Thérèse Laberge Samson, RD
Recipes by **Margot Brun Cornellier**

Your Health at Heart

Essential facts & tasty recipes

Translated by **Alison Lee Strayer**

Guy Saint-Jean
ÉDITEUR

Bibliothèque et Archives nationales du Québec and Library and Archives Canada cataloguing in publication

Laberge Samson, Thérèse
Your health at heart
Translation of: Manger de bon cœur.
Includes bibliographical references and index.
ISBN 978-2-89455-305-3
1. Cardiovascular system – Diseases. 2. Cardiovascular system – Diseases – Nutritional aspects.
3. Cardiovascular system – Diseases – Diet therapy – Recipes. I. Brun Cornellier, Margot. II. Title.
RC667.L3213 2009   616.1   C2008-942580-4

The Publisher gratefully acknowledges the financial aid of the Government of Canada through the Book Publishing Industry Development Program as well as the assistance received from SODEC for our publishing activities.

© Guy Saint-Jean Éditeur inc. 2009
Editing and translation: Alison Lee Strayer
Graphic Design: Christiane Séguin
Cover photograph: Getty images

Legal Deposit first quarter 2009
Bibliothèque Nationale du Québec and the National Library of Canada
ISBN 978-2-89455-305-3

GUY SAINT-JEAN ÉDITEUR INC.,
3154, boul. Industriel, Laval (Québec) Canada, H7L 4P7. Tel. (450) 663-1777. Fax: (450) 663-6666.
E-mail: info@saint-jean.editeur.com • Web: www.saint-jeanediteur.com

Printed and bound in Canada

Contents

Foreword

Your *Health at Heart* came to be as the result of an encounter between nutrition and fine cooking, the two main interests of the co-authors. In 1989, Madame Thérèse Laberge Samson, a nutrition and health-cuisine enthusiast, met with Madame Margot Brun Cornellier, a survivor of heart surgery, to teach her the basics of heart-friendly meal planning.

For years Madame Samson had dreamed of writing a book that would combine information on nutrition with healthy recipes. She discussed it with Madame Cornellier. Months passed, then one day Madame Cornellier contacted Madame Samson to say that she had modified 150 of her best recipes and ask if she would revise them. And this is how the adventure started. A first book was published in 1990, a second in 1997, and this third in 2009.

This incomparable book includes the best recipes from the first two books as well as an instructional section entitled "Your Guide to Healthy Eating", a sort of "user's manual" for individual cardiovascular health. This unique creation includes a series of charts that enable readers to determine their personal cardio health profile.

A word from the authors and collaborators

You care about health, so this book is for you. The section entitled "Your Guide to Healthy Eating" provides explanations that will support your initiatives for treatment and prevention, and introduces the basics of a healthy diet. Do you suffer from heart disease or diabetes? This book will prove invaluable in helping you change your dietary habits, one step at a time. You will discover recipes that are both healthy and delicious. Take the plunge, try out a few new recipes, new fruits, new vegetables…!

Remember the joys of old-style cooking, those dishes served at Christmas, Easter and birthdays? Those were days when the house was filled with delicious aromas of herbs and spices, and pots bubbled away for hours with recipes passed down for generations.

Today, things have changed; our lifestyles are different and our diets must sometimes be adapted to the requirements of one's own health. The hour of glory has arrived for "light-style" recipes and health-conscious cuisine. And we sincerely believe that health and pleasure can go hand-in-hand. The recipes in this book have been developed by a person who knows this from personal experience. Madame Margot Brun Cornellier once suffered from heart disease, and her husband was diabetic. She has always loved to cook and her reputation as a culinary wizard extends far beyond her family circle. Conventional dietary cuisine seemed to her too restrictive, so she put her chef's imagination to work, adapting her best recipes with the encouragement of her sister-in-law, Jeannine Cornellier, and nutritional advice from Thérèse Laberge Samson. Now it's your turn – get ready to SAVOUR this book!

Nutritionally yours,

Thérèse Laberge Samson, RD, co-author
Louise Gagnon, RD, M.Sc., collaborator
Odette Navratil, RD. M.Sc., collaborator

We remember the delicious food our mother prepared every day. And we really mean "every day" because the recipes that you will find in this book are the ones we enjoyed on a daily basis.

We rarely heard our mother say that she had run out of ideas for meals, for she was constantly inventing new recipes or modifying old ones. It was certainly not Margot who invented junk food! Without being complicated, her dishes were nicely presented and prepared with only the best ingredients.

We will always remember what our father said to our mother when he especially enjoyed one of her dishes: "Don't throw that recipe out!" Maybe it was hearing this phrase for almost forty years that inspired our mother to write three whole books of these recipes.

Another memory that comes to mind: when we were children, a friend of our father said to us: "You're lucky to have a mother who is such a good cook; when we come to eat at your house, it's like dining at the Château Frontenac." At such a young age, words like that leave quite an impression. We should add that Margot was the type of person who loved having visitors – whatever the weather, in sickness and in health. We think she acquired this from her own mother.

Even after we moved out and our father died, in 1999, our mother never lost her love of good cooking and having people over. Any occasion was an excuse for a good family dinner.

And today, Margot, you are no longer here. You left us just a little too soon to see and appreciate your final work.

We are proud of you and miss you very much.

François and Jean

Preface

In recent years, science has made spectacular advances in the diagnosis and treatment of heart disease and strokes. Nonetheless, cardiovascular illness remains the number one cause of death in this country, and this has become true of women as well as men.

And so, the battle is far from over. Eight out of ten adults in Canada would have to claim one or more risk factors for heart disease. That is far too many!

When we examine these factors more closely, we see that the majority can be controlled and even modified. Eating is one of those modifiable factors and plays a major role in cardiovascular health.

Adopting a healthy and varied diet can require a certain amount of discipline for people who have not acquired the habit in childhood, but it is well worth the effort. There is much evidence to prove that nourishing, balanced meals help reduce the risks of heart disease and stroke, maintain healthy weight, reduce high blood pressure and cholesterol, and control blood sugar levels.

To eat well every day is to take charge of your health.

Along with a varied selection of easy, nutritious recipes, *Your Health at Heart* offers a 'Teaching' section, a companion which will guide all your healthy dietary initiatives. The tasty dishes prepared by Margot Brun Cornellier, backed by a team of nutritionists, will remind you of home-cooking and introduce you to healthy foods from here and all over the world.

Cooking and eating well are pleasures that must be reclaimed – the healthy way.

Believe me, your heart with will thank you for it!

Dr. Jacques Genest
Cardiologist
Spokeperson for the Heart and Stroke Foundation of Québec

PART 1

Achieving optimum cardiovascular health

YOUR GUIDE TO HEALTHY EATING

Chapter 1 Introduction

You have just bought yourself a new recipe book because you want to improve your health. Oh yes, you'll discover new taste sensations, but eating healthily is a very big challenge!

In this guide to healthy eating, we will try to facilitate the process. In everyday language we will explain some of the information on diet and health that we receive from so many sources, not always knowing what to make of it. The guide has been designed with you in mind. The different sections will help you take charge of your diet, at your own rhythm, to maintain or improve your cardio health.

You may have wondered what causes cardiovascular disease. It is the result of a large number of conditions that we call risk factors. In Chapter 2 (p. 18), you will learn that they fall into two major categories: modifiable risk factors and non-modifiable risk factors. Next, by completing chart 1 (p. 18), you can identify your personal risk factors, and in chart 2 (p. 20) determine your risk level: low, moderate or high (with the help of your doctor). If you are wondering about your "target cholesterol level", chart 3 (p. 24) at Chapter 3 (p. 32) will help you identify which level corresponds to your risk profile.

Next, in Chapter 4 (p. 34), we will examine a recent concept, the metabolic syndrome. Increasingly recognized as an early warning sign of cardiovascular illness, metabolic syndrome affects a large segment of the population.

In Chapter 5 (p. 36), we will discuss the rules of healthy eating, more precisely, those outlined in *Eating Well with Canada's Food Guide*. We will also discuss energy or calorie balance. We know that when it comes to changing your diet, it isn't enough to simply acquire new knowledge. You have to apply the rules and stick to them, which requires motivation. In Chapter 6, (p. 38) we outline a new method that will help you determine your own level of motivation.

It is often difficult to begin and maintain this changing process without the support of a professional. Also in Chapter 6, we tell you how to contact a dietician/nutritionist, who is the person best qualified for the job of accompanying you.

In Chapter 7 (p. 40), we will discuss the nutrients and fatty acids most essential to cardiovascular health. Do you ever wonder about your energy (calorie) intake? In Chapter 8 (p. 58), you will find a simple method for calculating your daily requirement. Now that you know your risk level for cardiovascular disease, as well as your daily energy requirement, you can refer to chart 13 (p. 60) to calculate the number of daily required servings from each food group. These calculations are based on the recommendations of *Canada's Food Guide* and current data on the prevention and treatment of cardiovascular illness. You may have heard or read that certain nutrients such as antioxidants, soya protein, folic acid or B vitamins, and phytochemicals, flavonoids, plant stanols and sterols, can have a positive impact on cardiovascular health. In Chapter 9 (p. 62) we will provide you with information based on the most recent studies on these less-conventional nutrients. Are you diabetic and finding it difficult to follow the diet you've been given? If so, we've thought of you too. Each recipe in this book includes the number of dietary exchanges that correspond to each food group. Chapter 10 (p. 66) provides a clear explanation of the exchange system, a sample menu, and a word on artificial sweeteners. We have also provided a few useful addresses in case you require further information.

Since eating is a daily activity, and we sometimes run out of ideas, in Chapter 11 (p. 71) we have provided a few guidelines for menu-planning, and some pointers on grocery shopping as well as tips on reading labels on the packaging. Over the years you may have accumulated favorite recipes that you no longer make because they are too rich. Now there's no reason you have to give them up! Chapter 12 (p. 78) contains the secrets for transforming these recipes without sacrificing the flavors that you love! For those of you who like eating out, Chapter 13. (p. 82) shows you how to make enlightened choices in ordering from restaurant menus. Do you take anticoagulant medication, and have you been told to be careful about vitamin K? Chapter 14 (p. 86) answers your questions on the subject. If you have doubts about the quality of your diet, the "Self-evaluation and Self- instruction Guide" is for you (see Chapter 15 (p. 89). It provides a wealth of detailed information on healthy eating. Though it is aimed at the general public, we have not forgotten those of you who have been diagnosed with, or are at risk for cardiovascular illness.

This invaluable guide is designed for PROGRESSIVE individualized learning. It will help you become aware of the way you eat, and make changes, if necessary — in your own way and at your own rhythm.

We wish you the best of luck on your nutritional journey. Happy reading... and most of all, *bon appétit*!

Thérèse Laberge Samson, RD
Louise Gagnon, RD, M.Sc. and Odette Navratil, RD., M.Sc., collaborators

Chapter 2 Risk factors for cardiovascular disease

We cannot talk about cardiovascular disease (arteriosclerotic heart disease) without talking about prevention, because it is a kind of disease that develops *gradually*.

Poor eating habits are only one of the factors that accelerate the development of cardiovascular disease. As a group, they are called "risk factors" and some, like age, sex, heredity and ethnicity are *uncontrollable*. Others, however, are worth examining because they *can* be controlled. These include smoking, high blood pressure, dyslipidemias (anomalies in blood lipids or fats), diabetes, obesity and lifestyle factors (physical inactivity, a diet rich in saturated and trans fats which promotes the formation of fatty deposits in the arteries).

CHART 1

CALCULATING RISK FACTORS

Circle the one(s) that apply to you

NON MODIFIABLE RISK FACTORS	MODIFIABLE RISK FACTORS
Age*: Man over 55 years	Smoker
Menopausal woman	Dyslipidemia (irregularity of
Sex	the bloodlipids)
Heredity	Diabetes
Ethnicity	Obesity-overweight
	Lifestyle: Physically inactive
	Atherogenic diet

* Risk increases with age. If you are male and over the age of 55, or a menopausal woman, your age becomes a risk factor.

You may have heard about other, less-conventional risk factors such as: Lp(a), apo B , apo A1, etc. They are used as criteria in highly specific analyses performed by specialized clinics, often making it possible to detect cardiovascular illness at an earlier stage.

- You have started by determining which risk factors apply to you.
- Next, it is important to know your risk level in order to prevent or treat cardiovascular illness at an early stage.

If you are not diabetic and do not suffer from cardiovascular illness, the following exercise will help you determine your level of risk for cardiovascular disease in the next 10 years, that is:

- Low (less than 10 % risk) or
- Moderate (10 to 20 % risk) or
- High (greater than 20 % risk)

This can be calculated thanks to a 10-year coronary heart disease risk assessment model (see chart 2, p.20), developed by a group of Canadian researchers following an in-depth review of existing literature on cardiovascular illness. They established Clinical Practice Guidelines (2006) based on the global evaluation (measured by percentage) of a person's risk of developing a cardiovascular illness over a ten-year period. Diabetics or people with cardiovascular disease are automatically considered high risk. We strongly encourage you to do this calculation to gauge your level of personal risk. If you find the exercise too difficult or lack the required information, do not hesitate to ask for help from your G.P. or any other health professional.

To do this calculation, it is important to:

- locate your age group in chart 2
- know your cholesterol level, (ask your doctor)
- specify whether you are a smoker or non-smoker
- know your CT/HDL-C ratio (ask your doctor)
- know your systolic pressure (the top number in your blood pressure reading). For example, if your blood pressure is 120/80, 120 represents systolic pressure (ask your doctor)
- calculate the number of points that correspond to each risk factor
- circle the number of points corresponding to your profile
- add up the points for the five risk factors
- at the bottom of chart 2, locate the percentage corresponding to your total number of points
- with the help of chart 2, determine, your level of cardiovascular risk for the next 10 years: high (greater than 20 %), moderate (10 to 20 %) low (less than 10 %)

Chart 2

EVALUATING OVERALL RISK OF CARDIOVASCULAR DISEASE IN 10 YEARS

MEN		WOMEN	
Age	**Points**	**Age**	**Points**
20-34	-9	20-34	-7
35-39	-4	35-39	-3
40-44	0	40-44	0
45-49	3	45-49	3
50-54	6	50-54	6
55-59	8	55-59	8
60-64	10	60-64	10
65-69	11	65-69	11
70-74	12	70-74	14
75-79	13	75-79	16

TOTAL CHOLESTEROL (mmol/L)

Age	20-39	40-49	50-59	60-69	70-79
< 4,14	0	0	0	0	0
4,15-5,19	4	3	2	1	0
5,20-6,19	7	5	3	1	0
6,20-7,2	9	6	4	2	1
> 7,21	11	8	5	3	1

TOTAL CHOLESTEROL (mmol/L)

Age	20-39	40-49	50-59	60-69	70-79
< 4,14	0	0	0	0	0
4,15-5,19	4	3	2	1	1
5,20-6,19	8	6	4	2	1
6,20-7,2	11	8	5	3	2
> 7,21	13	10	7	4	2

SMOKER POINTS

Age	20-39	40-49	50-59	60-69	70-79
Non-smoker	0	0	0	0	0
Smoker	8	5	3	1	1

SMOKER POINTS

Age	20-39	40-49	50-59	60-69	70-79
Non-smoker	0	0	0	0	0
Smoker	9	7	4	2	1

MEN — CHOLESTEROL C-HDL

	Points
< 1,55	-1
1,30-1,54	0
1,04-1,29	1
> 1,04	2

WOMEN — CHOLESTEROL C-HDL

	Points
< 1,55	-1
1,30-1,54	0
1,04-1,29	1
> 1,04	2

EVALUATING OVERALL RISK OF CARDIOVASCULAR DISEASE IN 10 YEARS (suite)

MEN		
SYSTOLIC BLOOD PRESSURE		
	Points	
(mmHg)	**Untreated**	**Treated**
< 120	0	0
120-129	0	1
130-139	1	2
140-159	1	2
> 160	2	3

WOMEN		
SYSTOLIC BLOOD PRESSURE		
	Points	
(mmHg)	**Untreated**	**Treated**
< 120	0	0
120-129	1	3
130-139	2	4
140-159	3	5
> 160	4	6

TOTAL RISK POINTS	% RISK
0	1
1	1
2	1
3	1
4	1
5	2
6	2
7	3
8	4
9	5
10	6
11	8
12	10
13	12
14	16
15	20
16	25
> 17	> 30

TOTAL RISK POINTS	% RISK
9	1
9	1
10	1
11	1
12	1
13	2
14	2
15	3
16	4
17	5
18	6
19	8
20	11
21	14
22	17
23	22
24	27
> 25	> 30

My 10 year risk level is _____%.

My 10 year risk level is _____%.

If your family history is positive for cardiovascular illness (that is, there are people in your family who suffer from heart disease), your risk score must be multiplied by two.

Now that you know your risk level, together we will examine the two main categories of risk factors and try to understand their impact on cardiovascular health.

NON MODIFIABLE RISK FACTORS

They are those we can do nothing about but which still have to be taken into consideration:

Age

The risk of coronary disease increases with age and must be considered a risk factor in men over 45 years of age and menopausal women. The main reason for this is that older people are more subject than younger people to atherosclerosis (cholesterol deposits in the arteries).

Sex

The risk of coronary heart disease is higher for men over 55 years of age, and for menopausal women. Before menopause, women are less at risk than men.

Family history

A family history of cardiovascular illness (close family: parents, brother, sister) is considered a risk factor. Heredity factors must be evaluated with great care, especially when cardiovascular disease occurs in younger individuals and touches several members of the family. In this case, it may be necessary to go beyond immediate family members to determine the risk due to heredity.

Often positive heredity is associated with modifiable risk factors (see below). In short, heredity is a risk factor that must be considered when calculating your risk level.

Ethnicity

First Nations people and those of African or South Asian descent are more likely to have high blood pressure and diabetes and therefore, are at greater risk of heart disease and stroke than the general population.

MODIFIABLE RISK FACTORS

They are those that can be controlled:

Smoking

Smoking has many harmful effects. It reduces the supply of oxygen necessary for the heart's functioning; it causes fat to build up on the walls of the arteries, and contributes to the development of atherosclerosis; it causes the blood pressure to rise and the heart to beat faster. It is also responsible for chronic pulmonary illness, and cancer of the lungs and bladder. It is important to note that the weight people sometimes gain when they quit smoking is less harmful to health than smoking.

Smoking is associated with other risk factors as well. It increases the risk of cardiovascular illness and must be avoided at all cost.

Stress

Although stress can sometimes be a good thing, too much stress can be hazardous to your health and increase your risk of cardiovascular illness and stroke. The link between stress, heart disease and stroke is not entirely understood, but some individuals submitted to too much stress or stressed during long periods of time, may show higher cholesterol levels, an elevated blood pressure and seem to be more vulnerable to atherosclerosis (thickening of blood vessel walls).

Hypertension (high blood pressure)

Blood pressure is the force exerted by the blood on the walls of the arteries. Blood pressure that is consistently high forces the heart muscle to work harder. At the same time, it hastens the development of atherosclerosis in the arteries of the heart, brain, kidneys and eyes.

A diet high in salt can increase the blood pressure, so it is recommended that you limit your intake of salt and sodium-rich foods. That way, it will be easier to control your blood pressure and reduce the side effects sometimes associated with blood pressure medication. In Chapter 7 (p. 40) you will find an explanation of sodium, and dietary changes you can make to limit salt intake.

- **High cholesterol**

  High cholesterol is detected by means of a blood test called "a lipid profile". This test first reveals the total level of cholesterol (CT), but also gives information about so-called bad cholesterol (LDL-C), good cholesterol (HDL-C), triglycerides (TG) and the ratio of CT (total cholesterol)/HDL-C (good cholesterol atherogenic index).

- **Blood cholesterol**

  Blood cholesterol is a waxy substance produced by the body. Cholesterol is an essential component of the human organism, in which it fulfills a number of functions: it is essential to bile production, is a component of sex hormones, the adrenals and Vitamin D. However, when the level of cholesterol circulating in the blood exceeds a certain level, it must be very carefully monitored. It circulates through the blood vessels in the following forms: "good" cholesterol (HDL) and "bad" cholesterol (LDL) and (VLDL). No fat of any kind can freely circulate in the bloodstream. Fats require a transporter called lipoprotein (fat + protein). This fat-transporting protein can be of high density (HDL) or low density (LDL). See Chapter 3 "Lipid Profile" (p. 32), for the reference levels (normal levels) of cholesterol for your cardiovascular risk category. In Chapter 6 (p. 38), you will find recommendations for changing your eating habits in such a way as to reduce the amount of cholesterol you ingest from food. We invite you to fill out the "Self-Evaluation and Self-Instruction Guide" in Chapter 16 (p. 95).

- **HDL-C ("good cholesterol")**

  HDL-C ("good cholesterol") transports excess cholesterol to the liver, where it is transformed and eliminated. The higher your level of HDL-C, the better your chances of maintaining healthy arteries.

CHART 3

FACTORS INFLUENCING HDL-C LEVEL

HDL-C UP	DHDL-C DOWN
Heredity	Heredity
Sex (woman)	Sex (man)
Healthy weight	Obesity
Non-smoker	Smoker
Exercise	Sedentary
	High triglycerides
	Type 2 Diabetes
	Medication such as corticosteroids or beta-blockers

See Chapter 3 "Lipid Profile" (p. 32), for the target levels, or reference (normal) levels of HDL-C ("good cholesterol") for your cardiovascular risk category.

- **LDL-C ("bad cholesterol")**

Unlike HDL-C ("good cholesterol"), LDL-C, ("bad cholesterol"), comes from the liver and moves the cholesterol to the cells. It can be responsible for the build-up of cholesterol in the arteries when the level is too high, or its structure is modified, or the walls of the blood vessels are damaged. Most people with high cholesterol have a high level of mainly LDL-C ("bad cholesterol"). To bring the level down, your intake of saturated fats and trans fats must be reduced. In Chapter 3 (p. 32), you will find the target level (that is, the level to be attained), also known as the reference or normal level, of LDL-C ("bad cholesterol") for your cardiovascular risk category.

- **Triglycerides**

Triglycerides are a kind of "warehouse" for lipids or fats in the human body. Triglycerides "stockpile" excess calories, sugars and fats. They increase when a person is overweight or has a diet high in sugar, alcohol and fats. Exercise helps to diminish triglyceride levels. The target or reference level for triglycerides is less than 1.7.

Diabetes

Diabetes is the result of an imbalance in the body's ability to properly absorb sugar and starch. There are two kinds of diabetes: Type 1 Diabetes develops when the pancreas produces little or no insulin. This type of diabetes appears in childhood or adolescence. Insulin is a hormone responsible for maintaining the balance of glucose (sugar) in the blood, during and between meals. The absence of insulin is due to the gradual destruction of the pancreas by antibodies; it must be treated with medication and diet. In Type 2 Diabetes, insulin may be produced in low quantities, or in normal or even excessive quantities, but the body is unable to properly utilize it due to obesity, poor diet, disease or surgical removal of the pancreas, and the effects of certain medications. The resulting surplus of blood sugar contributes to the clogging of the arteries. Diabetes requires a very special approach to diet, which you may read about in further detail in Chapter 10 (p. 66) of this book.

Obesity

Before we discuss obesity and overweight, it is important to first talk about healthy weight. A person's healthy weight is calculated according to certain criteria, such as the Body Mass Index (BMI) or the waist measurement. Overweight and obesity are determined according to the same criteria.

- **Healthy body weight**

A healthy weight is not a specific weight you must try to attain or maintain. It is a range of realistic weights, established in relation to a variety of body types, and is above all a matter of health and well-being, not a question of appearance. How does one define the limits of obesity or thinness? Weight is an indicator of a person's risk of developing certain illnesses, but it is not the only risk factor. It is essential to consider other factors directly linked to health, such as family history and lifestyle. To evaluate the risk of weight-related illnesses, we use the Body Mass Index (BMI) and the waist measurement for reference.

To start with, it is important to:
- calculate your body mass with the help of chart 4 (p. 27).
- next, measure your waistline according to the suggested method.

Using chart 6 for reference (see p.28), you can easily determine if you are overweight or obese, according to the Body Mass Index.

- **The Body Mass Index (BMI)**

To determine if your weight presents a health risk, first you have to calculate your Body Mass Index (BMI). There are different ways of classifying body weight in terms of risk to health. The BMI takes account of your weight according to your height.

To find out whether your weight is in a safe range, all you have to do is:

1. Locate your height in the left-hand column of Chart 4 (p. 27).

2. On the same line, check whether your weight falls between the acceptable minimum and maximum.

You can also calculate your average healthy weight by adding the minimum and maximum weights (see Chart 4) corresponding to your height, and then dividing by two.

If your weight is below the minimum reference weight in the chart, it is important to determine why, e.g. small bone structure, illness, poor diet. Discuss it with your doctor. Underweight can expose you to a number of health problems.

If your weight is above the normal zone, you have a greater chance of developing health problems such as heart disease, high blood pressure, diabetes, arthrosis in

CHART 4

HEALTHY BODY WEIGHT — Method for evaluating

HEIGHT		MINIMUM WEIGHT		MAXIMUM WEIGHT	
Imperial	Metric	lb	kg	lb	kg
5 ft	1.52 m	101	46	127	56
5 ft 1 in	1.55 m	105	49	132	60
5 ft 2 in	1.58 m	110	50	136	62
5 ft 3 in	1.60 m	112	51	141	64
5 ft 4 in	1.64 m	119	54	147	67
5 ft 5 in	1.66 m	121	55	152	69
5 ft 6 in	1.68 m	123	56	156	71
5 ft 7 in	1.72 m	129	59	160	73
5 ft i 8 in	1.74 m	134	61	167	76
5 ft 9 in	1.76 m	136	62	169	77
5 ft 10 in	1.78 m	138	63	174	79
5 ft 11 in	1.81 m	144	65	180	82
6 ft	1.84 m	150	68	187	85
6 ft 1 in	1.86 m	154	70	191	87

1 kg = 2.2 lb

CHART 5

CALCULATING YOUR PERSONAL HEALTHY BODY WEIGHT

Your current weight	Your height	Your healthy weight range		Your healthy weight
		Minimum	Maximum	
_____	_____	_____	_____	_____

Weigh-in: once a week

Date:_____

Weight:_____

CHART 6

DETERMINING THE RISK OF ILLNESS BASED ON BMI (Body Mass Index)

Classification	Category BMI	Risk of developing health problems	My BMI	My risk level
Underweight	< 18.5	High	_____	_____
Normal weight	18.5-24.9	Low	_____	_____
Overweight	25.0-29.9	High	_____	_____
Obesity	> 30	Very high	_____	_____

Note: For persons 65 and over, the "normal" range for BMI is from 20 to 27.
Chart:
> : less than
< : greater than

the lower limbs, pain in the hips, knees and ankles. Obesity limits your quality of life, walking, travel... But the situation cannot be corrected overnight. We suggest that you give yourself time and proceed gradually – and do not hesitate to ask your doctor for help, for example, a referral for nutritional counseling.

It is important to remember that your BMI reading should be considered a more accurate indicator of your weight-loss goal than any particular weight you wish to attain.

You can also calculate your BMI using the following formula (please note that to use this evaluation method, your weight must be in kilograms and your height in meters)

BMI = Weight (kg) ÷ Height (m²)

Limitations of the BMI approach to weight evaluation

The BMI has certain limitations. It does not take account of fat distribution on the body. Moreover, it can lead to inaccurate classification for certain sectors of the population, for example:

- People who are naturally very slender and muscular;
- Very tall or very short people;
- People from certain ethnic or racial backgrounds;
- People over 65.

Please note that these charts for healthy weight and BMI do not apply to children.

Now use the below chart to determine whether you are overweight or not, according to your waist measurement.

The waist measurement

The waist measurement is an important health-risk indicator. It allows you to determine whether or not you are at risk in terms of fatty deposits in the abdominal region. Studies have shown that the *location* of surplus weight is an important element to consider in a health risk* evaluation. As a matter of fact, the accumulation of weight in the abdominal area is more harmful to health than if it occurs in the hips and thighs. Upper and lower limits for the waist measurement are determined according to sex:

CHART 7

THE WAIST MEASUREMENT METHOD

My waist measurement is

Upper limit

Men: waist measurement more than 102 cm (40 in)**   _____

Women: waist measurement more than 88 cm (35 in)**   _____

With a measuring tape, surround the waist between the last rib and the upper part of the pelvis.

**Persons of Chinese or South-Asian descent have different upper limits: men: more than 90 cm (35 po), women: more than 80 cm (32 po).

For a more specific evaluation of health risks, you can combine the BMI with the waist measurement. It sometimes happens that people with normal BMI have waist measurements in excess of established thresholds (see above), and vice versa.

Using both types of measurement, you will acquire a more precise idea of your weight-related health risks. Remember that the waist measurement and the BMI are only two of the existing tools for determining weight-related health risk. A health

---

* Risk of Type 2 Diabetes, dyslipidemias, hypertension and coronary heart disease. In excess of these figures, health risks are greater.

CHART 8

HEALTH RISK EVALUATION BASED ON BMI (Body Mass Index) AND WAIST MEASUREMENT

WAIST MEASUREMENT	NORMAL	OVERWEIGHT	OBESE
BMI:	(18.5-24.9)	(25.0-29.9)	(30 or more)
Less than 102 cm (men) Less than 88 cm (women)	Lesser risk	Increased risk	High risk
102 cm or more (men) 88 cm or more (women)	Increased risk	High risk	Very high risk

Circle the number that corresponds to your waist measurement: _____

Your risk level is _____.

professional is in a better position to evaluate your general state of health, taking account of lifestyle factors, family history, and other clinical variables.

All studies have shown that being even slightly overweight can put you at risk for cardiovascular illness, diabetes, hypertension and dyslipidemias. On the other hand, it has also been demonstrated that even a slight weight loss of 5 to 10% (4 kilos or 10 lbs) can be enough to reduce the risks of developing these illnesses, even though one's healthy weight is not attained.

Lifestyle

Lifestyle factors include physical activity level and nutrition. It has been demonstrated that physical inactivity and atherogenic diet have a devastating effect on cardiovascular health.

Physical inactivity is associated with a higher occurrence of cardiovascular illness. On the other hand, regular physical activity can improve your cardiovascular health. It helps decrease levels of LDL (bad cholesterol) and blood triglycerides, raises levels of HDL (good cholesterol), increases sensitivity of insulin and reduces hypertension and obesity. It also contributes to stress reduction, weight control, and promotes better sleep. It is important that the exercise be regular, the intensity and length of time depending on your individual capacity. It is recommended that you do at least 30 minutes of exercise per day, every day. Besides all the health benefits, you will feel great! We strongly recommend that you contact your local community health clinic to acquire a copy of *Canada's Physical Activity Guide to Healthy Active Living*. You can also consult the web site: www.guideap.com. This guide will help you find a program that corresponds to your needs and abilities.

Atherogenic diet: it has been clearly demonstrated that a diet high in calories, saturated fats, trans fats, concentrated sugars and salt has a negative impact on cardiovascular health. This kind of diet increases levels of LDL-C (bad cholesterol) and triglycerides in the blood, while decreasing HDL-C (good cholesterol), raising blood pressure and contributing to diabetes and obesity. A diet that is rich in fruits, vegetables, fibre and unsaturated fatty acids, has the exact opposite effect.

Together we have reviewed the different risk factors for cardiovascular illness. Using the risk factors chart, Chart 2 (p. 20), you have also determined your personal risk level:

Low (less than 10 % risk) _____

Or

Moderate (10 to 20 % risk) _____

Or

High (greater than 20 % risk) _____

Now we will take a look at the lipids profile and try to understand what it means.

Chapter 3 The lipid profile: target (reference) levels:

The lipid profile is a blood test performed on an empty stomach after a 10 to 12 hour fast. It gives you information on:

- CT (total cholesterol)
- LDL-C ("bad cholesterol")
- HDL-C ("good cholesterol")
- CT/HDL-C ratio
- Triglycerides

The target levels in the lipid profile (those to be attained, also called reference levels or normal levels) vary from one individual to the next, depending on whether you are high, moderate or low risk for cardiovascular disease. It is important to be very sure about your risk level, having filled out the chart in Chapter 2 (p. 18) of this book. Your family doctor can also help you, so do not hesitate to ask him or her about the results of your lipid profile and to explain its contents.

Because the target level for the lipid profile is established in terms of other risk factors, we have chosen to introduce it at this stage in the book. The elements of the lipid profile used to evaluate target levels for each risk category are as follows:

- LDL-C ("bad cholesterol")
- Ratio of CT (total cholesterol) to HDL-C ("good cholesterol")

CHART 9

RISK CATEGORIES AND TARGET BLOOD LIPID LEVELS

RISK LEVELS	TARGET LIPID LEVELS		
	LDL-C (mmol/L)		Ratio CT/HDL-C (mmol/L)
High * > 20% risk in 10 years or diabetes or cardiovascular illness	< 2.5	or	< 4.0
Moderate 10 to 20 % risk in ten years	< 3.5	or	< 5.0
Low < 10 % risk in 10 years	< 4.5	or	< 6.0

Key
> : greater than
< : less than
LDL-C: "bad cholesterol".
CT: total cholesterol.
HDL-C: good cholesterol.
Ratio: Total cholesterol is divided by the HDL-C.

Includes people with non-controlled cardiovascular illness, adult diabetics, people suffering from chronic kidney failure and those with a controlled cardiovascular illness.

My target level of LDL-C (bad cholesterol) is _____.
My target level of Ratio CT (cholesterol total/HDL-C ("good cholesterol") is _____.
My risk level is   high _____.
                   moderate _____.
                   low _____.

Please note that age is a major factor in risk calculation. A younger person could have a low 10-year risk estimate but still be at risk and require treatment.

Chapter 4 Metabolic syndrome

DEFINITION

Metabolic syndrome affects a greater and greater percentage of North Americans. Metabolic syndrome is not a specific illness, but a group of ailments, and is associated with poorly functioning metabolism. When detected and treated at an early stage, it helps prevent illnesses such as hypertension, Type 2 diabetes, dyslipidemias and cardiovascular illness. The syndrome is typified by a constellation of risk factors. The major elements of the syndrome are:

- obesity or excess abdominal fat;
- physical inactivity;
- genetic factors.

Metabolic syndrome is also closely associated with a metabolic disorder called *insulin resistance*, in which the cell's response to the normal action of insulin is defective. Overweight and physical inactivity trigger insulin resistance. The majority of people who display insulin resistance are abdominally obese (waist measurement above normal levels). The relationship between insulin resistance and all the metabolic risk factors is complex. A variety of risk factors are present in the metabolic syndrome; the ones listed below are generally considered most typical of this syndrome:

- Abdominal obesity (waist measurement that exceeds normal levels);
- Hypertension;
- Insulin resistance (slightly elevated blood sugar level);
- High level of blood triglycerides;
- Low levels of HDL-C (good cholesterol).

Three of these factors must be present in order to diagnose metabolic syndrome. People displaying the syndrome would be three times as likely to develop a cardiovascular disease, and four times as likely to develop diabetes.

TREATMENT

There are different ways of treating metabolic syndrome. The first approach is to modify the causes, that is, to treat obesity and physical inactivity in order to decrease the metabolic risk factors. It is strongly recommended to use this as your basic approach, with the second one as a complement.

The second approach is to directly treat metabolic risk factors, that is, hypertension, insulin resistance (elevated blood sugar) and dyslipidemia (high triglycerides and lowered HDL).

To know exactly where you stand in terms of metabolic syndrome, ask your doctor about your blood pressure, your fasting blood sugar level, your readings of HDL-C (good cholesterol) and triglycerides.

The treatment goals for metabolic syndrome are as follows:

CHART 10

GOALS TO ATTAIN IN TREATING METABOLIC SYNDROME

My current statistics:

WAIST MEASUREMENT (ABDOMINAL CIRCUMFERENCE):

Man	< 102 cm (40 in)	_____
Woman	< 88 cm (35 in)	_____
Blood pressure	< 120/80 mmHg	_____
Fasting blood sugar level	< 6.0 mmol/L	_____
LDL-C (bad cholesterol)	< 2.5 mmol/L	_____
HDL-C (good cholesterol)		
Man	> 1.0 mmol/L	_____
Woman	> 1.3 mmol/L	_____
Triglycerides	< 1.7 mmol/L	_____

As we will often mention throughout this book, when you evaluate your own statistical data and see that one of them is over or under the normal levels accepted, it is important to talk to your doctor about it. First you will need to change your diet, with the help of this book, and then ask your doctor to refer you to a dietician/nutritional specialist.

Chapter 5 Balanced diet

EATING WELL WITH CANADA'S FOOD GUIDE

In changing your eating habits as prevention or treatment of cardiovascular illness, you need to make sure that your diet is well-balanced. Consult the recommendations in *Canada's Food Guide* (the 2007 edition, entitled *Eating Well with Canada's Food Guide*).

Canada's Food Guide was designed to help Canadians make informed choices about their diets. Based in dietary science, this user-friendly guide outlines food choices that fulfill individual dietary needs, promoting health while decreasing the risks of chronic food-related illness. Foods are divided into four groups:

- vegetables and fruit;
- grain products;
- milk and alternatives;
- meat and alternatives.

Canada's Food Guide recommends a number of daily servings for each food group, based on age and gender. An optimum combination of food and exercise will help you feel better and maintain a healthy weight. It is important to vary your diet, making sure to include a lot of vegetables, fruit and grains. Choose low-fat dairy products, lean meats and two servings of fish per week, prepared with little or no fat. Consume salt, coffee and alcohol in moderation.

Eating is a pleasure. Food adds warmth and cheer to gatherings of family and friends. Food nourishes your body. It supplies the energy you need for all your daily activities. You do not need to deprive yourself of your favorite foods in order to stay healthy. But you do need to remember variety and moderation. And don't forget to take a look at *Canada's Food Guide* on line at: www.healthcanada.gc.ca/foodguide or contact your local community health clinic to acquire a copy.

ENERGY BALANCE

We often hear about "energy balance", but do we really know what it means? It simply refers to the relation between our consumption of food and liquids (calorie or energy intake) on one hand, and on the other hand, the expenditure of this energy (calories) for bodily functions (breathing, digesting and sleeping) and physical activity (calorie or energy expenditure).

Total energy intake must be sufficient to maintain a healthy weight and allow for variety in the daily diet. If we consume more calories than we need the imbalance translates into weight gain, regardless of the kind of food that has been consumed in excess. On the other hand, if we burn more calories that we take in, weight loss will result. Do you have questions about this subject? Does your weight concern you? You will find the answers to your questions in Chapter 2 (p. 18) of this book. Why not fill out the "Self-evaluation and Self-instruction Guide" in Chapter 16 (p. 95)? Or ask your family doctor to refer you to a dietician/nutritionist who will review your food profile with you. This nutritional specialist will guide you towards a diet that takes account of current recommendations for the treatment and prevention of cardiovascular disease, chapter 7 (p. 40) and support you in your weight-loss goals, if you so require.

Chapter 6 Modifying your eating habits

YOUR LEVEL OF MOTIVATION

Reading this book will allow you to acquire new knowledge and may make you want to change your eating habits, or even try out new recipes. In the past you may have tried to change some of your long-time eating habits but were unable to maintain the new ones. When you are trying to change a habit, your degree of motivation makes a big difference. We are often quite aware of how motivated (or unmotivated) we are, and that can be a trap when it comes to making changes. External factors such as responsibility for meal preparation, frequency of meals eaten in restaurants, and lack of time can seem like insurmountable obstacles. The number of changes you will make in your diet largely depends on your current eating habits and cardiovascular health.

It is more and more commonly recognized that before making a change, if we want

CHART 11

DETERMINING YOUR LEVEL OF MOTIVATION

WHICH OF THE FOLLOWING DESCRIBES YOUR LEVEL OF MOTIVATION?	YES or NO
Pre-contemplation: You deny (or do not believe) that your behavior is a problem. You do not see the advantages of changing this habit.	_____
Contemplation: You have mixed feelings about the advantages and disadvantages of changing your eating habits.	_____
Preparation: You are convinced of the advantages of changing your eating habits.	_____
Action: you are changing your behavior.	_____
Maintenance: you have sustained your change in behavior for 6 months since you first moved into action.	_____
Relapse: You transition back to your earlier, problematic behavior. But do not consider it failure. This stage is an integral part of the process and must be viewed as a learning experience. Use it to adopt protective measures against further relapse.	_____

to maintain that change, it is important to determine at what stage you are at in terms of your own motivation. Here are the stages outlined by the Prochaska method (Chart 11, p. 38), and some guidelines for calculating your personal motivation level, if you wish to do so.

If you only have a few changes to make and your motivation level is high, it is very likely that you will manage on your own. However, if you have major changes to make, do not hesitate to consult a dietician/nutritionist, who will:

- support your behavioral changes in a positive and effective manner.
- evaluate or check how motivated you are about making changes.
- help you boost your motivation and overcome barriers to change.
- support you when you move into action so that the action will be sustained.

The decision to change a habit is the result of a natural process that is carried out in steps over an extended period. Each step is the foundation for the following step. The role of the dietician/nutritionist is essentially to acknowledge, reinforce and facilitate your natural progression through the steps.

You can ask your family doctor to refer you to a dietician/nutritionist. If you are insured for private health care or treatments paid by your employer, it is important to check if nutritional counseling is reimbursed in part or in full.

Chapter 7 # Nutrients with direct impact on cardiovascular health

TYPES OF NUTRIENTS

In this section, we will discuss different food groups and dietary energy sources in terms of their impact on cardiovascular health:

- lipids: cholesterol, saturated fat, trans fat, polyunsaturated fat, Omega-3 fatty acids, monounsaturated fat;
- proteins;
- carbohydrates;
- fibre;
- salt;
- alcohol.

First we will describe each of these elements. Next we will discuss the daily recommended intake of each of the above (percentage of total intake), and other dietary recommendations. Numerous scientific studies have proven that nutrition plays an essential role in cardiovascular health.

Lipids or fats

Lipids, also called fats or fatty acids, are an essential energy source. One of their functions is to supply the organism with essential fatty acids and energy (calories). They also help the body absorb vitamins A, D, E and K. The main sources of lipids in our food are meat, poultry, fish, cheese, nuts and grains (sesame, sunflower, etc.), margarines, shortening, butter and oils.

Lipids or fats are found in different forms: cholesterol, polyunsaturated fat, Omega-3s, saturated fat, trans fat. As these words appear on most labels on the food we buy, and each of these fats play a different role in our diet, it is important to make a distinction between them.

Dietary recommendations

Whether your risk for cardiovascular disease is low, moderate or high, the total recommended quantity of fat is around 25 - 35% of your total daily energy intake.

HEALTHY WAYS OF COOKING MEAT, POULTRY AND FISH

METHOD	ADVICE	ADVANTAGES
Poached (cooked in liquid)	With the cooking liquid (water, milk, wine broth), let it get to boiling point but not actually boil.	Little or no added fat.
Sauté (cook at high heat with a small quantity of oil)	Quickly brown in a little olive oil (and stirring often.) Note: as soon as food changes color, it has generally lost some of its food value.	Rapid cooking preserves the nutrients and aromas of food.
Pan frying (quick frying on both sides, in a pan)	Use a non-stick pan or add a small quantity of fat. When using non-stick pans, cook over medium or low heat, because these pans do not hold up well in high heat.	Little or no added fat
Slow-cook (place a bit of liquid in a casserole and cook over low heat for several hours)	Remove visible fat. Inexpensive cuts may be used as slow cooking makes meat tender. You can brown food first in a little fat, if desired.	Requires little or no fat. Slow cooking brings out the flavor of food.
Steam (cook over boiling water)	Make sure the cover allows steam to escape, to prevent excess heat.	As water does not touch food, vitamins and other nutrients are preserved.
In 'papillotes' (cooked in oven, in tinfoil or parchment)	Add spices and fine herbs to develop aromas.	No added fat. Preserve flavors and nutrients.
Braising (slow cooking over low heat in a tightly-covered pot/casserole)	Do not add water. The water in the food condenses, sinks to the bottom and evaporates.	No added fat. Aromas and nutrients enrich cooking juices.

Meat, poultry and fish

- Choose lean cuts of meat, i. e: meats with little or no "marbling" of fat (do not hesitate to ask your butcher).
- Trim fat from meat and poultry; before cooking, remove all visible fat and all skin from poultry.
- Remove fat from ground meat for use in casseroles by running cold water over it after cooking, and before adding other ingredients.
- Cook meats without adding fat, or use only a small quantity of fat for browning, grilling, roasting or sautéing.
- Slightly reduce the quantity of meat in recipes, and increase the quantity of vegetables.
- Once in awhile, replace some or all of the meat you intend to use with shredded tofu or legumes (lentils, kidney beans, etc).
- Eat fish at least twice a week.

Choosing the best sources of fat

Margarines

The margarine/butter debate has been going on for years and will keep on going, because it affects two huge food industries and has major economic impact. Butter is a primary source of saturated fat. Thus for spreading on bread, it should be replaced with non-hydrogenated margarine.

But how do we choose the right margarine? Select a soft, non-hydrogenated kind, preferably canola oil or olive oil-based (these are the oils with the highest percentage of monounsaturated fat), or a kind without trans fat and whose saturated fat is less than 1.5 fat/serving.

Oils

It is recommended that you choose vegetable oils like olive or canola oil. For pan frying, choose olive oil (in small quantities) over other oils because it is more stable when heated. For a salad dressing or cooked food, canola oil is recommended for its higher levels of essential fatty acids.

CHART 12

ILLUSTRATION OF LABEL ON A TUB OF MARGARINE

Example of a Nutrition Facts chart on a tub of margarine, for a recommended serving of 10 g (2 tsp):

NUTRITION FACTS
Par 2 tsp (10g)/for 2 tsp.

Content	% Daily intake
Calories / Calories 70 Cal	
Total Fat / Lipides 8.0 g	12%
Saturated / saturés 1 g	
+Trans / trans 0 g	5%
Polyunsaturated / polyinsaturés 2.5 g	
Omega-6 / oméga-6 2 g	
Omega-3 / oméga-3 0.6 g	
Monounsaturated / monoinsaturés 3.5 g	
Cholesterol / Cholestérol 0 mg	0%
Sodium / Sodium 70 mg	3%
Total Carbohydrate/ Glucides	0%
Dietary Fibre / Fibres alimentaires 0 g	0%
Sugars / Sucres 0 g	
Protein / Protéines 0 g	
Vitamin A / Vitamine A	10%
Vitamin C / Vitamine C	0%
Calcium / Calcium	0%
Iron / Fer	0%
Vitamin D / Vitamine D	30%
Vitamin E / Vitamine E	15%

Eggs

Limit your intake of egg yolks to two to three a week, for they are a major source of cholesterol. Egg whites and egg substitutes can be consumed as often as desired.

Milk and dairy products

Opt for fat-reduced dairy products: 2%, 1% or skim milk, cheese with less than 20% butter fat. You can find that information in the "% M.F." (% butter fat) reading on the label.

Salad dressings, dips, sauces and soups

- Replace fat-rich salad dressings with a few teaspoons of olive oil and wine or balsamic vinegar, seasoned with fine herbs.
- Is your favorite commercial dressing one of the creamy kinds? Reduce its fat content with light mayonnaise or plain yogourt.
- In dips, replace mayonnaise or cream with plain yogourt.
- Store-bought mayonnaise can be replaced by tofu mayonnaise (whip 1/2 of a 225 g square of tofu, with 2 tbsp. lemon juice, 2 tbsp. olive oil, 2 tsp. Dijon mustard, 1tsp honey) which contains 2 g of fat per tbsp., compared with 11 g for store-bought mayonnaise.
- Prepare sauces with 1% milk or concentrated skim milk instead of cream; or use half milk-half cream for more taste and a creamier texture (this also goes for creamy soups, e.g. potage).
- To remove fat from sauces and broths, put them in the refrigerator and skim off the fat that forms at the surface.
- Season vegetables with lemon juice or fine herbs rather than butter.

Pastries, baked goods and muffins

- It is possible to reduce one-third of the fat in recipes without affecting texture or taste.
- To make even lower-fat baked goods, replace up to one-half of the oil, margarine or butter with unsweetened apple sauce.
- Some of the whole eggs can be replaced with egg whites (for 2 eggs, use 1 whole egg and 1 egg white).

The different types of fat

- **Dietary cholesterol**

There has been so much said about the harmful effects of cholesterol that it is hard to believe that it is an element naturally present in the human body, essential to its functioning. In fact, a distinction must be made between *dietary cholesterol*, which is found in all food of animal origin, and *blood cholesterol*, which is naturally present in the human body.

Dietary cholesterol is a substance similar to fat. It is exclusively found in food of animal origin (egg yolks, liver and other organ meats, shrimp and the muscle fibre in meat). A high level of blood cholesterol, as we mentioned in Chapter 2 (p. 18), can result from high dietary cholesterol and fat. Thus it is recommended to limit your consumption of food with a high cholesterol content.

Dietary recommendations

The recommended intake of dietary cholesterol varies according to your risk of cardiovascular illness: less than 300 mg for low risk, less than 200 mg for moderate or high risk.

- **Saturated fats**

Saturated fats can generally be recognized by the fact that they are solid at room temperature. They are principally found in fats of animal origin such as butter, suet, cheese, cream, non-skim milk and meat, as well as certain fats of vegetable origin such as palm or coconut oil and shortening. These fats raise the level of "bad" blood cholesterol (total cholesterol and LDL-C), so they should be consumed in limited quantities.

Dietary recommendations

Whether your cardiovascular risk level is moderate or high, the recommended quantity of saturated fat is less than 7% of daily energy intake. If your risk level is low, the recommended quantity is less than 10% of total daily energy.

- **Trans fats**

Trans fat raises the bad cholesterol level and reduces the good cholesterol level.

It is formed through a process of hydrogenation, used by the food industry to make products last longer and give them a better taste, appearance and texture. That is why we find the highest incidence of dietary trans fat in commercial products. Since January 2006, Health Canada has required companies to make a separate entry for trans fat content on the Nutrition Facts table on the packaging, and all manufacturers have had to observe this requirement since 2008.

However, it applies only to certain pre-packaged products and not food served in restaurants.

Dietary recommendations

Whether your risk level for cardiovascular illness is low, moderate or high, the recommended quantity of trans fat is below 1% of daily energy intake.

Practical advice for reducing your daily trans fat intake
- Use non-hydrogenated oils, preferably canola or olive oil. For deep frying, do not use canola oil, and never re-use oils more than two or three times.
- Carefully check the list of ingredients on labels and avoid those containing the words: hydrogenated and/or partially hydrogenated vegetable oil or hydrogenated fat, because these products contain trans fat.
- Limit as much as possible the following commercial products: fried potatoes, doughnuts, sugar-rich cookies, and crackers because they are high in trans fat (check the Nutrition Facts chart on packaging).
- Limit your intake of saturated fat in your daily diet. If your diet is low in saturated fat, you are probably consuming little trans fat.
- When eating in restaurants, avoid ordering fried food, not only because it is high in fat but also because it contains hydrogenated fat and therefore is high in trans fat.
- Avoid commercial shortenings and all commercial food products fried in oil, such as french fries, chicken or fish sticks, etc., because they contain trans fat.

In summary:
It is very important to consider the types of fats you eat. Most people with high blood cholesterol would be well advised to reduce their consumption of food products containing saturated fat, trans fat and high cholesterol content.

- **Polyunsaturated fats**

Polyunsaturated fats can be identified by their relative softness and greasy appearance at room temperature or when refrigerated. They are essentially found in products of vegetable origin (safflower, sunflower and corn oil, soft margarine made with these vegetable oils) and in fatty fish. When consumed in moderation, replacing saturated fats, they tend to bring down your level of blood cholesterol.

Dietary recommendations

Whether your risk of cardiovascular illness is low, moderate or high, the recommended quantity of polyunsaturated fat must not exceed 10 % of your daily total energy intake.

Certain foods are high in polyunsaturated fatty acids and can be consumed on an occasional basis:

- soya, safflower, sunflower, corn and sesame oil;
- flax, pumpkin and sunflower seeds;
- walnuts, pine nuts;
- fish (trout, salmon, sardines, etc.).
- non hydrogenated soft margarine

- **Omega-3 fatty acids**

Omega-3 fatty acids, of vegetable origin, are essential fatty acids belonging to the polyunsaturated fat family. They are called "essential" because they are necessary to the development and functioning of the human body, which cannot manufacture them itself. Thus it is important to consume a sufficient quantity of these in food. Omega-3s of marine origin have a very well-defined role in cardiovascular health. They contribute to the dilation of blood vessels, a decrease in the formation of blood clots, the lowering of blood pressure and the level of blood triglycerides. They have an anti-inflammatory effect and are also useful in the prevention of other chronic illnesses.

Omega-3s come from two sources:

Vegetable

- Provide ALA (alpha-linolenic acid). ALA is an essential fatty acid.
- Help reduce the ratio Omega-6/ Omega-3 (to promote the efficiency of the Omega-3s).

Animal (marine origin)
- Provide EPA and DHA (eicosapentaenoic and docosahexaeonic acids).
- Possess the cardioprotective properties that people seek from Omega-3s.

Sources of vegetable origin (ALA)	Sources of marine origin (EPA/DHA)
Flax	Fatty fish:
Canola	Herring
Hemp	Salmon
Walnuts	Rainbow trout
	Mackerel
	Sardines
	Canned tuna
	Halibut

(Lean fish and seafood contain lower quantities)

Dietary recommendations
It is suggested that you consume:
- 2 to 5 servings (90 g/serving) per week of fatty fish, as mentioned above, as well as:
- Daily consumption of Omega-3 of vegetable origin e.g. 2 tsp. ground flax seeds, 1 tbsp. Canola oil or 60 ml (1/4 cup) walnuts.

Practical advice for daily consumption of Omega-3s
How can you apply these recommendations on a daily basis? Why not try some of the fish recipes in this manual? Here are a few tips about cooking fish.
- It is important to cook fish at a high temperature (200-220 °C /400-450 °F) for a short period.
- Calculate 5 to 10 minutes per 2.5 cm (1 inch) of thickness at the fleshiest part of the fish.
- Fish can be baked in the oven, barbecued, steamed and poached. Never defrost fish before cooking, that way the flesh will remain firmer; instead, double the cooking time.
- Enhance the flavor of fish with herbs, lime or lemon juice, or balsamic vinegar.
It is important to consume Omega-3s of vegetable origin every day, such as walnuts

(add to cereal, yogourt and salads), flax seeds (add to yogourt) and canola oil (use in cooked dishes).

Fish or supplements?
Fish should be your first choice. As a matter of fact, it seems that eating two servings of fatty fish per week results in a 23% reduction in mortality due to cardiovascular illness, and eating it more than five times a week reduces the risk by 38%.

Moreover, the nutritional value of fish is far higher than that of a supplement. Fish contains proteins with anti-inflammatory properties, as well as selenium, a powerful antioxidant not found in Omega-3 capsules. Finally, replacing a meat meal with a fish meal is also very good for your health, for meat contains more saturated fat than fish. If you are thinking of taking a supplement, it is important to check with a nutritionist whether it is useful to do so.

- **Monounsaturated fats**

These fats do not increase blood cholesterol. Consuming monounsaturated fats instead of saturated fats helps reduce the level of bad blood cholesterol (LDL) without reducing the level of good cholesterol (HDL).

Dietary recommendations
Whether your level of cardiovascular illness is low, moderate or high, the recommended quantity of monounsaturated fat should not exceed 20% of your total daily energy intake.

Monounsaturated fatty acids are found in the following foods:
- olive and canola oil;
- avocados;
- hazelnuts, almonds, peanuts, pistachio nuts, pecans, sesame seeds;
- natural peanut or almond butter;
- soft non hydrogenated margarine made from a monounsaturated oil.

Practical advice for using monounsaturated fats in your daily diet
When you must use fat in cooking, olive oil is recommended because it is more stable when heated.

Here it should be mentioned that your doctor may find it necessary to prescribe an antilipemic medication (to modify the level of lipids in your blood). It is scientifically recognized that if you follow the appropriate dietary recommendations, the effects of this kind of medication are intensified, and if your diet does not comply with recommendations, the effects of the medication may be counteracted. Do not hesitate to discuss it with your doctor, nutritionist or pharmacist.

Proteins

Types of proteins

Proteins are, in some sense, the building blocks for the organism. The body uses them to form and maintain muscle mass and fight infection. Proteins are of animal origin (meat, poultry, fish, eggs, dairy products), or vegetable origin (legumes, nuts and grains). Animal proteins are whole foods, easily assimilated by the organism; vegetable proteins, on the other hand, are incomplete and must be combined with other vegetable proteins to be effectively absorbed. Combined, they "complement" or complete each other, which is why we talk about protein complementarity.

But the combining of vegetable proteins cannot be left to chance. They can be combined in three ways:

- grains and dairy products,
- or legumes and grain products,
- or legumes, nuts and/or seeds.

They must be combined in this way on the same day. You may find it easier to combine them in the same meal, with a dairy or meat product, or in the following manner:

Legume (250 ml/1 cup) + grain products (250 ml/1 cup) or bread (1 slice)
Sample menu: Comforting pea soup (250 ml/1 cup) (p. 121), Celeriac salad (p. 216), Curried rice (250 ml/1 cup) (p. 128), Berry delight (p. 246)

Legume (250 ml/1 cup) + nuts or seeds (85 ml/1/3 cup)
Sample menu: Comforting pea soup (250 ml/1 cup) (p. 121), Four seasons salad (p. 221), Summer almond fruit treat (p. 245)

It is also recommended that you eat meals that do not contain meat, that is to replace meat once or twice a week with a meal based on:

- legumes, for example pea soup, lentils, kidney beans, chick pea salad, legume loaf, vegepaté, etc., without forgetting to combine them with complementary foods on the same day (nuts, grain products, seeds);
- egg whites, or limiting the quantity of egg yolks to two per week;
- cheese, choosing the fat-reduced kind (less than 20% M.F.).

Dietary recommendations

The intake of proteins, whether vegetable or animal, should be between 10 and 15% of your total energy intake, whether your level of risk for cardiovascular illness is low, moderate or high.

- *Canada's Food Guide* recommends two to three servings per day.
- The recommended serving per meal is 75 g (2 $^1/_2$ oz). This quantity satisfies the basic protein requirement.

Carbohydrates

Carbohydrates, also known as starches or sugars, are the main source of energy in the human body

Types of carbohydrates

There are two categories of carbohydrates:

- simple sugars: these supply quick energy because they reach the bloodstream in a very short time. The main sources are concentrated sugars (white and brown sugar, honey, molasses, maple or other syrups, jam, candy), fruits and fruit juice, certain vegetables, milk and dairy products;
- complex sugars: foods that contain complex sugars do not have the sweet taste of those that contain simple sugars, for their main source is starch. Complex sugars can be found in flour, vegetable starch (from potato, corn, tapioca, etc.), bread, grain products, rice, potatoes, pasta and vegetables.

Because they are digested more slowly, complex sugars provide longer-lasting energy. Thus it is important to increase the complex sugars in your daily menu by consuming more bread and grains (preferably whole grains) and certain simple sugars, such as fruit and vegetables. As these whole foods provide an excellent source of fibre, they help lower blood cholesterol and ensure better intestinal functioning.

Dietary recommendations

Whether you are low, moderate or high risk for cardiovascular disease, the recommended quantity of carbohydrates is 50 to 60% of total daily energy intake. For those with high triglycerides, the recommended quantity of carbohydrates (sugar) should not exceed 50% of total energy intake.

Whether your risk for cardiovascular illness is low, moderate or high, it is important to consume most of your carbohydrates (sugar) from fibre-rich products such as grains and whole-grain breads, vegetables, fruit and low-fat or fat-free dairy products.

Practical advice for reducing simple or concentrated sugar in your daily diet

- We suggest that you consume the following only once in awhile: concentrated sugars such as brown and white sugar, fructose, molasses, maple or corn syrup, honey, caramel, jams and other spreads, marmalades, chocolate milk, soft drinks and fruit punches, candy, chocolate, doughnuts, flavored jellies, commercial puddings, sugary cereal, dried and candied fruit.
- In most recipes, the quantity of sugar or brown sugar can be cut in half without affecting the taste or texture of the final product.
- White and brown sugar can be replaced with an equal quantity of date puree with a little water added to make it creamy. What is the advantage of doing this? Dates provide fibre and vitamins.
- In recipes, the quantity of honey or molasses can be cut in half, substituting pineapple or apple juice, and adding 5 minutes to the cooking time.
- Choose breakfast cereals that are not only fibre-rich (4-6 g or more/serving) but also low in sugar (6 g or less, or 10 g or less if they contain fruit).

Practical advice for increasing the quantity of complex sugars in your daily diet
Complex sugars (from fruit, vegetables and cereal products) are more nourishing.

- To increase your intake of complex sugars, we suggest you follow the recommendations in *Eating Well with Canada's Food Guide*, increasing the quantity of bread and grain products to 5 or more servings per day. This group includes a variety of foods based on fibre-rich whole-grain flour.
- Increase the quantity of fruit and vegetables you eat daily.
- Replace pastries and baked goods with fruit. Home-made cakes and pastries can be

consumed in moderation if they are made with non-saturated fats, minimal quantities of sugar and egg yolks, and as often as possible with fruit.

Dietary fibre
Types of fibre
Dietary fibre is a substance that is not, or is only slightly digested by the digestive system. Fibre is essential to the functioning of the intestines and can help bring down blood cholesterol. It provides a feeling of fullness, which can help with appetite and weight control.

Dietary fibre is divided into two main categories:
- Soluble fibre (which forms a gel when mixed with water) can help bring down the level of bad (LDL) cholesterol and the level of blood glucose in a diabetic person.
- Insoluble fibre (which does not dissolve in water) increases the volume of stools and makes intestinal functioning more regular. It helps prevent constipation and other ailments of the digestive system.

Dietary recommendations
The recommended quantity of fibre for adults is 25 to 35 g per day.

To help you achieve this daily intake, we have provided the levels of soluble fibre for certain foods (below). When you do your grocery shopping, check nutrition facts charts. They will tell you how much fibre products contain and make it easier to calculate your daily intake.

The main sources of soluble fibre are:

SOURCES	serving	# g fibre/serving
Psyllium powder	5 ml/1 tsp.	3 g
Kellogg's All Bran Buds with psyllium fibre	85 ml ($^1/_3$ cup)	3 g
Oatmeal or cooked oat bran	125ml ($^1/_2$ cup)	1.5 g
Cooked barley	200 ml ($^3/_4$ cup)	1.5 g
Orange	1 large or 4 fresh apricots	2 g
Fruit	1 medium-sized	1 g

Vegetables such as asparagus, broccoli, carrots, Brussels sprouts, turnip, green beans, onions, sweet potato, frozen green peas	125ml ($1/3$ cup)	1-2 g
Legumes, e.g. lima beans, white, red or black beans, chick peas	125ml ($1/2$ cup)	1 to 3 g
Metamucil	1 envelope	13g

The main sources of insoluble fibre are:

SOURCES

Bran and whole grain products, such as whole-grain cereal, rye
Vegetables and fruit
Nuts and grains
Legumes.

For the quantity of fibre contained by each of these foods, carefully check the nutrition facts chart on the packaging.

Practical advice for increasing your daily fibre intake

- Choose breakfast cereals containing 3 g or less fibre, 5 g or less sugar, and 10 g or less sugar if the cereal contains fruit.
- Choose food bars containing 2 g or more of fibre, and 2 g or less of saturated and trans fat.
- Choose crackers containing 2 g or more of fibre, and 2 g or less of saturated or trans fat.
- In recipes for baked goods, replace half or more of the white flour with whole-wheat flour. This will help increase the fibre quantity.
- Choose whole-wheat or multigrain pasta and brown rice with 4 g or more fibre.
- Sprinkle salads with walnuts, soy beans or sesame seeds instead of croutons and bacon bits.
- Add fibre to casseroles or puddings and yogourt by sprinkling them with oat bran or cereal with psyllium.

- Serve vegetables at meals; you will find numerous recipes in this manual for soups, salads, etc.
- Why not add lentils, chick peas, kidney beans to your soups and spaghetti sauces?

Salt (sodium choloride)

The sodium in salt affects blood pressure, and most of us consume more salt than our organism requires.

Dietary Recommendations

It is a good idea to reduce your sodium intake to the recommended level of 2.3 g or less a day (2300 mg). This is the equivalent of a little more than 1 tsp. of salt.

To reduce daily sodium intake to the recommended quantity of 2300 mg (2.3 g) or 1 tsp. per day, you may need to make a few changes in your eating habits. Here are a few tips.

Practical advice for reducing daily salt intake
- Avoid salting food during meals.
- When cooking, salt food in moderation, always taste before adding salt. Certain foods, such as tomato juice and cheese, already contain a lot of salt, enough to add taste to dishes without your having to add more. We often have little control over our salt intake, due to the overuse of salt and other sodium compounds in the food processing industry. Therefore it is important to check the Nutrition Facts chart for the quantity of sodium per serving, or the list of other ingredients on the packaging. On this list, sodium may appear under the following names: sodium, sodium chloride, sodium bicarbonate, monosodium glutamate, baking powder, table salt, sea salt, vegetable salt, garlic salt, and all other ingredients including the word *sodium*.
- Gradually replace salt with herbs and spices, garlic and onion powder, garlic, lemon, flavored vinegars or tabasco to enhance the flavors of your home-made dishes. It will allow you to discover and develop new tastes.
- Reduce your consumption of commercially prepared food. Soup concentrates, cold cuts, smoked or salt-cured food, salt-based seasonings, marinades, snack bar food, salty cocktail snacks and most mineral waters all contain a lot of salt and must be consumed in moderation.

In the "Recipe" section of this book, the quantity of sodium has been included with every recipe. This complies with the standards of the DASH Eating Plan (Dietary Approaches to Stop Hypertension).

Alcohol

We are well aware that alcohol brings pleasure when it is consumed in moderation. We also know that the subject of alcohol and the treatment of cardiovascular disease is very controversial! Let us review the benefits and adverse effects of alcohol with regards to cardiovascular disease, as well as a few precise recommendations based on current research.

Benefits:

- An increase in good cholesterol (HDL); however, physical exercise has the same effect, without negative side effects.
- Alcohol or other components of alcoholic beverages, such as resveratrol, are purported to prevent the agglomeration of blood platelets that causes blood clots; however, low doses of aspirin have the same effect, without side effects, if administered with care.
- Flavonoids and other antioxidants found in red wine are purported to lower the risk of cardiovascular illness; however, some of these components can be found in other foods, such as grapes or grape juice.

Adverse effects:

- Contributing factor in increasing blood triglycerides.
- Contributing factor in increasing blood pressure.
- Contributing factor in heart failure.
- Increases calorie intake.
- Contributing factor in absenteeism at the workplace, car accidents, digestive and neurological illness.
- Strictly forbidden for persons suffering from alcohol dependence, for the above reasons and for overall individual health.

Recommendations

In light of the above facts, and if you agree with what has been said about the adverse effects of alcohol, we advise you to discuss the subject with your doctor. He or she can evaluate the benefits and risks in terms of your own personal health.

If you are allowed alcohol, it is recommended that you do not exceed the following quantities:

- 1 or 2 servings/day for men
- 1 serving/day for women

1 serving is equal to:

- 375 ml (12 oz) beer
- 150 ml (5 oz) dry wine
- 90 ml (3 oz) dessert wine or porto
- 45 ml (1 ^{1}/$_2$ oz) spirits

Chapter 8   Personalizing your needs profile

QUICK CALCULATIONS OF ENERGY REQUIREMENTS BASED ON LEVELS OF PHYSICAL ACTIVITY

At this point of the book, it is logical for you to wonder about your own personal energy (calorie) requirements. Though it will not replace a visit to a dietician/nutritionist, we have a quick-calculation method to suggest.

1. Determine your healthy weight in Chapter 2 (p. 18). To convert your weight from pounds to kilos, divide your weight by 2.2.

2. Multiply this result by:

33 calories if you do no physical activity;

38 calories if you are moderately active (about 20 minutes of exercise 3 times a week);

44 calories if you are very active (training for competition).

For example, if your healthy body weight is 70 kg and you are moderately active, your energy requirements for one day are:

70 kg X 38 calories = 2660 calories per day.

I weigh _____ kg X _____ calories (according to my level of activity) = _____ calories/day

QUICK CALCULATION METHOD FOR PROTEIN, CARBOHYDRATE AND FAT REQUIREMENTS

To find out your daily requirements for proteins, carbohydrates and fats, which are the most important nutrients (macronutrients), responsible for your daily energy (calorie) intake, use the following method. For each of these nutrients, you must respect the percentages recommended in Chapter 7, that is 10 to 15% for proteins, 50 to 60% for carbohydrates and 25 to 35% for lipids.

Calculate 10 to 15% of your daily required energy (calorie) intake for proteins and divide the total by 4 (because a gram of protein provides 4 calories). This will give you the number of recommended daily grams of protein.

Example:

2660 calories X 15% = 399 calories

399 calories / 4 = 100 g protein/day

My personalized calculation of required protein per day

Number of calories _____ X 15 % = _____ calories

Number of calories _____ / 4 = _____ g proteins/day.

Calculate 55 to 60%/day of your energy (calorie) requirement for carbohydrates and divide the total by 4 (because a gram of proteins provides 4 calories). This will give you the number of recommended daily grams of carbohydrate.

Example:

2660 calories X 55% = 1466 calories

1466 calories /4 = 367 g carbohydrates/day.

My personalized calculation of required carbohydrates/day

Number of calories _____ X 55 % = _____

Number of calories _____ / 4   = _____.

Calculate 30 to 35 % of your daily energy (calorie) requirement for lipids and divide the total by 9 (because a gram of lipids provides 9 calories). This will give you the number of recommended daily grams of lipids.

Example:

2660 calories X 30 % = 798 calories

798 calories / 9 = 89 g lipids/day

My personalized calculation of required lipids/day

Number of calories _____ X 30% = _____

Number of calories _____ / 9 = _____.

To summarize, if you weigh 70 kg, your organism needs 2660 calories daily, distributed as follows: 100 g protein, 366 g carbohydrates and 89 g of lipids.

You have determined your energy requirements using the quick-calculation method, and now you know your protein, carbohydrate and lipid requirements, but how do we convert these figures into numbers of daily servings for each food group?

Chart 13 below is based on the nutritional and energy requirements of a person with a moderate to high risk level for cardiovascular illness.

Choose the number of calories closest to your daily requirement and you will obtain the number of daily servings from each food group that you need for a balanced diet.

If you have consulted Chapter 3 of this book and established that your risk level is low, you can determine your daily number of servings with the help of *Canada's Food Guide*, which very clearly indicates the number of daily servings for each food group according to age and sex.

CHART 13

NUMBER OF RECOMMENDED SERVINGS FOR EACH FOOD GROUP BASED ON A LEVEL OF MODERATE TO HIGH RISK OF CARDIOVASCULAR ILLNESS

	MODERATE LEVEL OF RISK					HIGH LEVEL OF RISK				
kCal	2500	2000	1800	1600	1200	2500	2000	1800	1600	1200
Meat	3	2 1/2	2 1/2	2 1/2	2 1/2	3	2 1/2	2 1/2	2 1/2	2
Eggs/wk	2	2	2	2	2	1	1	1	1	1
Dairy products	4	3	3	3	3	4	3	3	3	2
Fat	8	6	5	4	3	7	6	5	4	3
Breads & Grains	12	10	8	7	4	12	10	8	7	4
Vegetables	5	3	3	3	3	5	3	3	3	3
Fruit	5	5	4	4	4	7	5	5	4	4

- Prevention: 1% or 2% milk
- Treatment: Milk 0% M.F.
- 1 additional egg may be added if for cooking
- For all food groups, it is important to respect the serving size recommended in *Eating Well with Canada's Food Guide*.

Results

I calculated my energy (calorie) requirement at _____ (see beginning of section # 8).

My number of servings/day is:

Meat: _____ servings.

Eggs: _____ servings.

Dairy products: _____ servings.

Fat: _____ servings.

Bread: _____ servings.

Grains: _____ servings.

Vegetables: _____ servings.

Fruit: _____ servings.

Chapter 9 # Evolution in cardiovascular nutrition

OTHER NUTRITIONAL FACTORS

Studies show that other nutrients, besides the ones we have already mentioned, can have a bearing on cardiovascular disease. In certain regions, the Mediterranean for example, where the diet is rich in fruits, vegetables, whole grains, sea fish and unsaturated fats, the risk of cardiovascular disease seems to be lower. On the other hand, in regions like Eastern Europe and Russia, the risk of cardiovascular disease is much higher. These observations have led researchers to wonder what elements of the Mediterranean diet could have a positive effect on cardiovascular health. Here are the main ones:

Omega-3 fatty acids

Please see Chapter 7 (p. 40) for further information on this subject.

Folic acid, vitamin B6 and B12

These elements play a role in the metabolism (transformation) of a certain amino acid (homocysteine) which is purported to have an effect on cardiovascular health. Research has not come up with enough conclusive evidence to recommend vitamin supplements for folic acid and these two B-vitamins. It is strongly recommended that you follow the guidelines in *Eating Well with Canada's Food Guide* (you can acquire a copy through your local community health clinic) or the model outlined in Chart 13.

This way, you will be assured that you are absorbing a sufficient quantity of these elements through your food.

Antioxidants

Antioxidants include vitamins such vitamin C, vitamin E, beta-carotene, bioflavonoids and selenium, which are purported to play a role in decreasing the oxidation (ageing) of cells and thereby reduce the risks of cardiovascular illness. Research has demonstrated the importance of raising the RDA (recommended daily allowance) of vitamins C and E, for both men and women. *Eating Well with Canada's Food Guide* takes these increases into account. In conclusion, it is unnecessary to take vitamin supplements. If your risk level is low, just follow the recommendations in *Canada's Food Guide* and your nutritional needs will be met. If your risk level is moderate or high, follow the recommendations in Chart 13 (p. 60).

Plant stanols and sterols

Plant sterols are natural components of cellular membranes in plants. They are not produced by the human body, but can only come from food. They are found in vegetable oils, regular margarine, vegetables, sunflower seeds, fruit, vegetables, and grain products, but only in very small quantities. For plant sterols to bring down the levels of cholesterol (C-total and LDL, so-called bad cholesterol), they must be taken in large quantities. Plant sterols offer additional support to patients who do not respond well to medication. They are added to normal or light margarine and salad dressings. However, this type of plant sterol enrichment is not allowed in Canada, due to potential side effects.

Soya protein

In the Orient, soya has been a basic food forever. The Japanese consume approximately 55 g (2 oz) of soya protein per day and statistics reveal half as many deaths related to cardiovascular disease in their country as Americans, whose consumption of soya products averages 5 g per day. The effect of soya protein on cardiac health has been studied for about 25 years. The last major studies showed a very modest decrease: a 3% reduction of bad cholesterol (LDL) and an approximately 6% reduction of triglycerides, if one consumes 50 g (2 oz) of soya protein per day. As for the increase in good cholesterol (HDL), the effect of soya protein is negligible. In short, experts estimate that the direct effects of soya proteins in the daily diet are minimal. However, if they replace a diet rich in animal fat, saturated fat and cholesterol, soya products (tofu, soya protein, soya butter, tofu burgers), high in fibre, vitamins and minerals, they can be beneficial to cardiovascular health.

Sources of soya protein:
- Soya milk
- Cooked soy beans (30 g for 1 cup)

- Soy nuts (5 g par 30 g)
- Soya cheese (4 g par 20 g)
- Soy-based frozen desserts (2 g per 100 ml)
- Soy-based meat substitutes (10 g per 100 g)
- Soy breakfast sausages (11 g per 50 g)
- Firm tofu (10-16 g per 100 g)

The consumption of 25 to 50 g (1 to 2 oz) of soya protein per day as a replacement for products of animal origin has proven to be an effective and safe way for causing a (modest) reduction in LDL-C ("bad cholesterol") and triglycerides.

Natural products

Several other so-called natural products (garlic, hawthorn, red yeast rice, policosanol, coenzyme 10, carnitine, artichoke, chitosan) are also used by some people to prevent or treat cardiovascular disease. These are not miracle products, in spite of what they claim (these claims are without scientific basis). Though some may prove to have certain benefits, it is important to talk to your doctor, dietician/nutritionist or pharmacist if you plan to try these products. For instance, you should discuss the combined effects of several natural products taken concurrently (at normal dosage), the interactions between pharmaceutical and natural products, especially for those which had few or no clinical studies done to prove their effectiveness, not withstanding the possibility that some of them might have certain toxic side effects. In short, these products are not recommended by health professionals.

Nutrigenomics

We thought we would very briefly mention a new field that combines nutrition and genetics. Experts predict that rapid progress in genetics will revolutionize preventive medicine, nutritional therapy and nutritional policy in the public health sector. This new field is called nutrigenomics. It studies the structure, regulation and role of genes in metabolism, and how nutrients work. It also examines the hereditary factors that condition the way people respond to nutrients and other natural components of food. In the near future, we may expect health professionals to analyse their patients' genetic constitution, predict their future health, issue personalized recommendations for diet, lifestyle and medication, and prescribe custom-designed treatments. Research in nutrigenomics already shows enormous potential for the prevention and treatment of chronic illness (including cardiovascular disease).

Chapter 10 # Diabetes

NUTRITIONAL NEEDS

If you are diabetic, your nutritional needs are similar to those of the general population. However, you must take care to eat a balanced diet with an appropriate distribution of proteins, carbohydrates (sugars) and lipids (fat). Diet planning, which is usually done by a dietician/nutritionist, takes account of several factors, such as daily habits, personal tastes, activity level, and prescription medications.

A personalized plan divides food into seven categories according to its protein, carbohydrate and lipid content. The seven groups are:

- fruit
- vegetables
- grain products
- dairy products
- meat and alternatives
- fats
- food with added sugar

Each group includes several equivalents, called "exchanges" or "choices". These terms refer to a measured quantity of a certain type of food that can be replaced by another from the same group. This system can be used to plan meals for the entire family, adapting serving sizes to individual requirements.

Using the exchange system

- Ask your dietician/nutritionist to draw up your daily eating plan (see example p. 67) and provide you with a sample menu. Only these professionals can draw up an eating plan that takes account of your dietary needs, depending on age, size, bone structure, gender and activity level. Other factors to be taken into consideration include personal taste, dietary habits, medication (tablets and insulin), various conditions linked to diabetes such as hypertension (high blood pressure), cardiac problems and dyslipidemias (changes in levels of blood lipids: cholesterol, triglycerides).

- Familiarize yourself with the various food groups and their recommended quantities in your eating plan.
- Use your eating plan at meal time to choose the appropriate number of exchanges for each food group.
- The exchange system offers a list of the most common foods in each food group. That is why certain foods are not included on the list. You can consume these unlisted foods as long as you know their carbohydrate content, because then you will know how to include them in your eating plan. To determine the content of carbohydrates and other nutrients in a particular commercial product, read the nutrition facts chart on packaging. Since dietary fibre has no effect on the level of blood glucose and is included in the total carbohydrates indicated on the label, it must be subtracted from the total carbohydrates if the product contains 5 g or more of fiber per serving. This is the case for most vegetables, as well as certain grain products that are rich in fibre.

CHART 14

SAMPLE DAILY MEAL PLAN

NUMBER OF EXCHANGES

	Morning	Snack	Noon	Snack	Evening	Snack	Daily total
Fruit	_____	_____	_____	_____	_____	_____	_____
Vegetables	_____	_____	_____	_____	_____	_____	_____
Grain products	_____	_____	_____	_____	_____	_____	_____
Dairy products	_____	_____	_____	_____	_____	_____	_____
Meat	_____	_____	_____	_____	_____	_____	_____
Food with added sugar	_____	_____	_____	_____	_____	_____	_____
Fats	_____	_____	_____	_____	_____	_____	_____

By following your eating plan, you will have a balanced diet and maximize your chances of controlling your blood sugar levels. We suggest that you:

- Eat according to your eating plan.
- Eat all the meals (and snacks, if applicable) that have been planned.
- Avoid changing the time at which you eat food containing carbohydrates because they have a direct impact on your blood sugar level. For example, avoid eating

an extra piece of bread in the morning and then omit it at noon.

- Eat meals (and snacks, if applicable) at the same time each day, when possible.
- Vary the foods in the same food group (for example, eat different kinds of fruit and vegetables),
- Notify your dietician/nutritionist if any significant changes occur in your physical activity level, or medication, general state of health, weight or appetite. Do not hesitate to ask about anything concerning your diet.
- Pay special attention to serving sizes. To begin with, we recommend that you weigh your food. Gradually you will develop a good idea of the serving size simply by looking at it. After that, you need only weigh your food occasionally to make sure your eyes are not playing tricks on you!

Make sure that your dietician/nutritionist gave you a list of foods for each of the seven food groups, along with your daily eating plan. We will look at this below in the section entitled "Possible exchanges for each of the seven food groups". Each serving on the list represents one exchange in the food group in question. For example: 125 ml (1/2 cup) of pasta = 1 starch exchange.

Possible changes for each of the seven food groups

Fruit: 1 exchange = 1 whole fresh fruit
1/2 grapefruit, 1/2 banana
125 ml (1/2 cup) fruit: puréed, fresh and in sections, or canned (drained)
125 ml (1/2 cup) unsweetened fruit juice or
2 to 3 dried fruits

Vegetables: 1 exchange = 125 ml (1/2 cup) vegetables: fresh, cooked or canned

Grain products   1 exchange = 1 slice of bread
125 ml (1/2 cup) cooked cereal
175 ml (5 oz) dry cereal
1 potato, plain
125 ml (1/2 cup) pureed potato
125 ml (1/2 cup) cooked pasta or rice
4 crackers, risks or melba toast

		125 ml (½ cup) cooked vegetables
		250 ml (1 cup) soup with pasta
Dairy products:	1 exchange =	125 ml (½ cup) milk
		125 ml (½ cup) plain yogourt
Meat:	1 exchange =	30 g (1 oz) cooked meat or chicken or fish
		1 egg 30 g (1 oz) low-fat cheese
		1 tbsp. peanut butter
Fats:	1 exchange =	1 tsp.margarine
		2 tsp. mayonnaise
		1 tbsp. home-made salad dressing
		1 tbsp. home-made sauce
Food with	4 exchanges =	1 slice lemon pie (⅙ of a 9 in. pie)
added sugar	4 exchanges =	1 slice of chocolate cake without icing
		(¹⁄₁₀ of a 9 in. cake)

Using the exchange system in recipes from this book

You have no doubt noticed that each recipe in this book provides you with the numbers of dietary exchanges.

> **Sample menu created with the recipes in this book with an illustration of the exchanges:**
>
> Cream of zucchini soup (p. 114) = ½ bread exchange, 1 vegetable exchange
> Beef brochettes (p. 153) = 3 meat exchanges, ½ fat exchange, 1 vegetable exchange
> Rice 125 ml (½ cup) = 1 bread exchange
> Orange-glazed carrots (p. 133) = 2 vegetable exchanges
> Mango-lime mousse (p. 247) = 1 fruit exchange
> 2 plain cookies = ½ bread exchange
> 250 ml (1 cup) milk = 2 milk exchanges

Sugars and artificial sweeteners

In people who are diabetic, the most common sugars such as white and brown sugar, honey and syrups, can cause a rapid rise in blood sugar. Therefore they must be limited as much as possible and replaced in certain recipes, if the taste of sugar is necessary, by an artificial sweetener. But sugar does more than just make food taste sweet; it also helps it brown, and grow light and crispy. As for sweeteners, they all have their advantages and disadvantages. Aspartame tastes like sugar, but loses its taste when used in cooking. Other liquid sweeteners are stable when used in cooking but unlike sugar, they do not make food crispy and golden. The granulated sweeteners are a combination of artificial sugar and natural sugar, such as lactose or dextrose. As sugar is indispensable in certain recipes, a small quantity may be permitted: about 1 tsp. per meal and 3 tsp. a day. Here are a few tips to make the calculation easier:

    1 cup (250 ml) = 48 tsp.
    1/2 cup (125 ml) = 24 tsp.
    1/3 cup (80 ml) = 16 tsp.
    1/4 cup (60 ml) = 12 tsp.

Sugar calculation

Example: If a recipe requires 80 ml (1/3 cup) of sugar for 12 servings, you can calculate the amount of sugar per serving as follows:

    1/3 cup = 16 tsp.
    16 tsp. sugar divided by 12 servings = approximately 1 tsp./serving

The Canadian Diabetes Association recommends that you do not consume more than 3 to 4 envelopes of sugar per day, or 6 to 8 tsp. of granulated sweetener. The dessert recipes in this book are prepared with Splenda. Used in equal quantities, it has the same sweetening value as sugar. Sweeteners are a temporary solution for those who find it difficult to adapt to a less sweet taste. If this is your case, try to make it your goal to become gradually accustomed to a less sugary taste and appreciate the natural flavors of food.

Chapter 11 Menu-planning and grocery chopping

MENU-PLANNING

Planning your menus for the week will help you avoid too many trips to the grocery store. It may also incite you to try new recipes by ensuring that you have all the necessary ingredients on hand. Here are a few suggestions for planning your weekly menus:

- Check the supermarket circulars. They will give you ideas for adding variety to your menus and also save you money.
- Plan your weekly menus based on the specials. In every meal, include foods from the four groups outlined in *Canada's Food Guide*. Think about harmonizing the colors and flavors.
- Choose your recipes.
- Make a list of the food items the recipes require.
- Make an inventory of food items you already have at home.
- Make your shopping list.
- Do your grocery shopping, reading labels carefully. Remember that good nutrition begins with food shopping. If you do not buy foods you should avoid, you will not be able to eat them at home!

UNDERSTANDING LABELS

Here you are at the supermarket. But how to know what to choose? How to make sense of all the labels? Here, we will try to make the task easier by explaining the information you will find on labels. We suggest that you:

- read this section of the book carefully;
- make separate photocopies of Charts 15, 16 and 17 (pages 73, 74, 76);
- make a special "learning trip" to the supermarket, taking your charts and familiarizing yourself with the "vocabulary" of labels;
- think about having charts 15 and 17 (pages 73, 76) coated in plastic and bring them with you when you shop for food.

Since we have been eating three meals a day for many years, isn't it worth spending a few hours to learn how to shop for food with health in mind? Once you have done that, grocery shopping can be accomplished in no time at all! It is strongly recommended not to go food shopping on an empty stomach; be sure to eat a healthy snack before leaving.

The labels on food packaging are an indispensable tool for helping you choose groceries. Five main elements appear on these labels: nutrient claims; the health claim; the *Health Check* logo (on certain products); the nutrition facts chart, and the list of ingredients.

The Nutrient Claim

The Nutrient Claim is a statement regulated by Health Canada that serves to highlight the nutritional characteristics of foods. It is optional and found on the labels for only certain foods. It normally appears on the front of packaging. However, we must understand its meaning in order to properly evaluate the product's food value. At page 73 you will find a chart illustrating the main nutrient claims with their meaning.

Health claims

The nutritional labeling chart on food can now include health claims. These indicate the relationship between diet and certain illnesses. In order to include health claims, the food must comply with strict and well-established criteria; moreover, the wording of these claims is standardized. For example, the health claims concerning heart disease read as follows:

"A diet low in saturated and trans fat reduces risk of heart disease. (Name of food) is low in saturated fat and trans fat."

"A diet rich in potassium and low in sodium reduces risk of high blood pressure, a risk factor for stroke and heart disease (Name of food) is a good source of potassium and is sodium free."

The *Health Check* logo

Health Check was developed by the Heart and Stroke Foundation as a resource for helping Canadians make healthy food choices. In concrete terms, it is a logo accompanied by an explanatory message combined with the "nutrition facts" table for all participating products (participation is voluntary). The nutrient criteria implemented by the program comply with the ones found in *Eating Well with Canada's Food Guide*. The same criteria determine whether a food product is eligible for the program or not. For more information on *Health Check*, visit their web site at: http://www.healthcheck.org.

CHART 15

LIST OF DIFFERENT NUTRIENT CLAIMS AND THEIR MEANING

NUTRIENT CLAIMS	MEANING
Without added sugar/ unsweetened	The food product contains no added sweeteners such as sugar, honey, molasses, fruit juice, fructose, etc. This does not mean that the product contains no carbohydrates but that it may contain sugars that are part of the food product, such as food starches or lactose.
Low fat	The product contains 3 g or less fat/serving.
Low in saturated fat	The product contains 2 g or less saturated fat and trans fat combined per serving.
Cholesterol free	The product contains less than 2 mg cholesterol/serving and must be low in saturated fat. This term does not mean that the food contains no fat; in fact, it could be high in fat and calories.
Salt free/sodium free	The product contains less than 5 mg of sodium/serving.
Low salt/low sodium	The product contains 25% less salt than the original version and no more than 140 mg sodium/serving.
Source of fibre	The product contains at least 2 g of fibre/serving.

The Nutrition Facts chart

The Nutrition Facts chart has been obligatory on most pre-packaged foods since December 2005, with the exception of:

- Fresh fruit and vegetables

- Raw meat, poultry, fish and seafood
- Food prepared in the store, such as: baked goods, sausages and salads.
- Food containing very few nutrients: coffee beans, tea leaves and spices
- Alcoholic beverages

The Nutrition Facts chart has three goals:

- To help you choose the food you need.
- To allow you to choose between similar products.
- To identify foods that contain (or do not contain) certain nutrients.

Now let us try and understand based on the example given in Chart 16:

(1) Specific quantity or serving; you must always adapt the serving size indicated on the label to the serving actually consumed; do this in order to compare two similar food products.

(2) Quantity of each of the 13 essential nutrients contained in the product per portion.

CHART 16

SAMPLE OF A NUTRITION FACTS CHART

NUTRITION FACTS
(1) Per 125 ml (87 g)

(2) Amount	(4) % daily value
(3) Calories　80	
(3) Fat　0.5 g	(4) 1%
(3) saturated　0 g	
(3) + trans　0 g	
(3) Cholesterol　0 mg	
(3) Sodium　0 mg	
(3) Carbohydrate　18 mg	
(3) Fibre　2 g	
(3) Sugars	
(3) Protein	
(3) Vitamin A	
(3) Vitamin C	
(3) Calcium	
(3) Iron	

(3) 13 essential nutrients.

(4) For most of the essential nutrients, figures are based on the recommended daily allowance for adults. The chart allows you to check whether a food product contains more or less of a given nutrient. It is based on a daily energy intake of around 2000 calories. It is important to compare the amount of sodium contained by different food products.

Remember that your sodium intake should be less than 2300 mg/day. Certain Daily Value percentages (% DV) allow us to identify whether a food product is "low" or "high" in certain nutrients:

- Saturated fat and trans fat: a product with a % DV of 10% or less is considered to be "low" in these nutrients.
- Fat, sodium and cholesterol: a product with a % DV of 5% or less is considered to be "low" in these nutrients.
- Fibre, iron, calcium: a product with a % DV of 15% or more is considered to be "high" in these nutrients.

You will tell me it is impossible to remember all these things at the supermarket. And you are right!

That is why we have designed our "Selection criteria for healthy food purchases", an indispensable resource that we encourage you to photocopy, have coated in plastic, slip into your wallet and consult on your "learning trip" to the supermarket, and all future shopping expeditions.

As we noted earlier, there is no nutrition facts chart on packaging for fresh meat and fish. For meat, here is a list of recommended lean cuts to be consumed on a regular basis: extra lean ground meat, round, loin, sirloin, filet, butterfly cut (breasts), escalope (scallops), skinless chicken breast. Fat must be removed before cooking. Other cuts not mentioned here may be consumed on an occasional basis. For fish, check the list of recommendations in Chapter 7 (p. 40) to make sure you are eating high in omega-3s.

The ingredients list

A food label can be full of surprises... for example, did you know that sugar, fat and salt in food go by many different names? Here is a list:

- sugars: fructose, sucrose, lactose, maltose, dextrose/dextrine, inverted sugars, sugar, honey or molasses.

CHART 17

SELECTION CRITERIA FOR HEALTHY FOOD PURCHASES

| | | FAT | | SODIUM | CARBOHYDRATE | | PROTEIN |
	Total	saturated	trans		Fibre	Sugars	
Bread **1 slice (50 g)**			5 % or less	480 mg or less	2 g and more (> 8% DV)		
Grains **30 g**		2 g or less (< 10% DV)	5% or less	480 mg or less	3 g or more (> 8% DV)	6 g or less	
Cookies **30 g**		2 g or less (< 10% DV)	5% or less	480 mg or less		6 g or less	
Crackers **20 to 30 g**	3 g or less	2 g or less (> 5% DV)	5 % or less	300 mg or less	2 g or more (> 8% DV)		
Cereal bars		2 g or less (> 10% DV)	5% or less	480 mg or less	2 g or more (> 8% DV)		
Pasta **85 g dry** **or 215 g cooked**				480 mg or less	4 g or more		
Frozen dinners **215 to 285 g**	10g and less (< 15% DV)	2 g and less (< 10% DV)	5% or less (< 30% DV)	720 mg and less			10 g and more
Commercial soups **250 ml**	3 g or less (< 5 % DV)		5 % or less	650 mg or less			
Milk **1 cup (250 ml)**	2% or less			240 mg or less			
Yogourt **175 g**	2% or less			480 mg or less			
Cheese **30 g**	2% or less			480 mg or less			
Frozen desserts	3 g or less		5% or less	480 mg or less		minimum	

- fat: glycerides, monoglycerides, esters (glycerol, shortening, hydrogenated vegetable oils, phospholipids, palm oil or palm kernel oil.
- salt: brine, sodium bicarbonate, monosodium glutamate (sodium, Accent, sea, kelp, soya sauce).

Ingredients are listed in descending order of weight. Foods in which one of the terms above is listed as a first or second ingredient should be consumed in moderation because they can considerably increase your daily intake of sugar, fat and salt.

This chart contains the most usual ingredients and is based on the Heart and stroke Foundation's *Health Check* program. If you wish to obtain further information, please visit the Foundation's web site at www.healthcheck.org, under *nutrition information*. Please do not hesitate to print it and take it with you whenever you go shopping for food. It is a perfect tool to learn to make the right choices.

Chapter 12 # Modifying your recipes

WORK METHOD

You are now ready to discover new recipes! When we buy a new recipe book, we flip through it, try a few recipes and then often put the book aside. If you want to take better advantage of your investment, why not consider some of the following tips?

- Start by trying one new recipe a week. Write a check mark beside the ones that turn out a success.
- Continue at this rhythm and little by little, you will change your way of eating.
- Now that you are familiar with nutritional labeling, you may compare the food value of each recipe. Do not hesitate to use it!
- If you have questions, why not treat yourself to a consultation with a dietician/nutritionist who will be able to answer all your questions and also guide you towards a tasty and healthy diet.
- To help you modify your recipes, see Chart 18 for a few suggestions for substitutions.

If a recipe does not appeal to you, adapt it to your own taste. You will no doubt notice that some of the recipes in this book are similar to your favorite dishes but have replaced, reduced or completely eliminated the butter, sugar or salt. Take note of these modifications and apply them to your own family recipes. Here, as an example (p. 80), is a recipe modified by Madame Cornellier. Read it carefully, and then it will be your turn to adapt some of the recipes you love!

Did you know that it is possible to take courses in healthy cooking? These could be particularly helpful to you if:

- you are still hesitating about taking charge of your diet;
- you have a personalized plan for dietary modification but have lost the motivation to continue;
- you have been cooking for years and have run out of ideas;
- you have never cooked and would like to take over some of the cooking or at least help prepare meals;
- you are committed to the prevention of coronary heart disease;
- you are unable to modify your own recipes.

CHART 18

INGREDIENT SUBSTITUTIONS TO ADAPT YOUR RECIPES

You can replace	With	In
Sour cream	Light sour cream, plain yogourt or cottage cheese 1 to 2 tbsp. lemon juice, light ricotta or Dama or quark, mixture of yogourt and ricotta	Dips, dressings, Chinese fondue sauce
Mayonnaise	Light mayonnaise, mixture of yogourt and ricotta	Dips, dressings, Chinese fondu sauce
Whole milk	Skim milk, 1 or 2%	Béchamel sauce, pudding, custard
15 or 35% Cream	Milk plus a starchy vegetable (potato, squash or corn), milk and pasta or grains (rice, barley ...) or cornstarch or potato starch	Potage (cream soup)
Whipped cream	250 ml (1 cup) light ricotta + 3 tbsp. plain yogourt + 2 tbsp. sugar. Ricotta whipped in mixture + fruit juice + honey + essence to taste	Dessert Icing for cakes
Butter, lard or shortening	Non hydrogenated margarine, canola or safflower oil	Cookies, cakes, muffins
Shortening or lard	Non hydrogenated margarine put in freezer for 30 minutes	Pie crust
1 egg	2 egg whites or 1 egg white + 1 tsp. vegetable oil	Cookies, cakes, muffins, crêpes
Egg yolk used as thickener	Corn or potato starch	Sauce
Cheese high in butter fat	Cheese with under 20 g fat	Broiled cheese dishes, pizza, lasagne
Chocolate	Carob	Desserts
Store-bought salad dressing	Home-made salad dressing: olive or canola oil, cider or balsamic vinegar, lemon juice	Salads
Quantity of fat required by recipe	Reduce to a third of the quantity required by the original recipe.	Muffins (60 ml or 1/4 cup fat for 12 muffins)
Pepperoni	Chicken, tuna or vegetables only	Pizza

CHART 19

COMPARISON OF INGREDIENTS BETWEEN A TRADITIONAL AND A MODIFIED RECIPE

ORIGINAL RECIPE	MODIFIED RECIPE
Beef bourguignon	**Beef bourguignon**
	(Margot Brun Cornellier)
6 SERVINGS	6 SERVINGS
1 kg (2 lb) beef, shoulder or round	**1 kg (2 lb) very lean beef in cubes**
4 slices of fat salt lard	**1 tbsp. olive oil**
60 ml (¼ cup) flour	60 ml (¼ cup) flour
1 tsp. salt	1 tsp. salt
¼ tsp. pepper	¼ tsp. pepper
1 leek	3 chopped green onions
¼ tsp. thyme	¼ tsp. thyme
60 ml (¼ cup) chopped parsley	60 ml (¼ cup) chopped parsley
2 minced cloves of garlic	2 minced cloves of garlic
250 ml (1 cup) dry red wine	250 ml (1 cup) dry red wine
250 ml (1 cup) carrot cut in rounds	250 ml (1 cup) carrot cut in rounds
250 ml (1 cup) pearl onions	250 ml (1 cup) pearl onions
250 ml (1 cup) small fresh mushrooms	250 ml (1 cup) small fresh mushrooms
2 tbsp. butter	**250 ml (1 cup) home-made chicken broth (see recipe p. 113)**

You can find out how to enroll in healthy cooking courses by contacting the dietary division of your hospital, the Heart and Stroke Foundation, your community health clinic or your regional school board.

CHART 20

COMPARISON OF NUTRITION FACTS BETWEEN A TRADITIONAL AND A MODIFIED RECIPE

ORIGINAL RECIPE (6 servings)	Amount	% DV	MODIFIED RECIPE (6 servings)	Amount	% DV
Calories	465		Calories	360	
Fat	25 g	39%	Fat	14 g	23%
Saturated	12 g	62%	Saturated	4.5 g	24%
+ Trans	0.1 g		+ Trans	0 g	
Polyunsaturated	2 g		Polyunsaturated	1 g	
Omega-6	1.7 g		Omega-6	0.8 g	
Omega-3 (ALA)	0.4 g		Omega-3 (ALA)	0.1 g	
Omega-3 (EPA+DHA)	0 g		Omega-3 (EPA+DHA)	0 g	
Monounsaturated	12 g		Monounsaturated	6 g	
Cholesterol	113 mg	38%	Cholesterol	822 mg	28%
Sodium	639 mg	27%	Sodium	531 mg	23%
Potassium	1022 mg	30%	Potassium	1051 mg	31%
Carbohydrate	12 g	4%	Carbohydrate	11 g	4%
Fibre	1.5 g	7%	Fibre	1 g	
Sugar	3 g		Sugar	3 g	
Protein	39 g		Protein	39 g	
Vitamin A		19%	Vitamin A		14%
Vitamin C		14%	Vitamin C		12%
Calcium		4%	Calcium		4%
Iron		31%	Iron		31%
Vitamin D		40%	Vitamin D		27%
Vitamin E		5%	Vitamin E		5%
Vitamin K		23%			

Chapter 13   # Eating out

INTRODUCTION

The frenzied pace of life today means we eat in restaurants more often. Restaurants offer us a range of foods to satisfy the most demanding palates. Whether you are dining out with friends or business associates, or simply in a hurry, it is possible to enjoy restaurant cuisine while sticking to a healthy eating plan. Most restaurants post their menu near the entrance, which allows you to check whether the food suits your requirements. You can also phone ahead to find out what is on the day's menu. Certainly, if you eat out only once a week or less, you can treat yourself to your favorite dish, even if it does not conform to your healthy eating plan.

GENERAL ADVICE FOR MAKING WISE CHOICES

Before dinner drinks

If you are obligated to avoid alcohol, go for mineral water with a twist of lemon, vegetable or tomato juice, or a 0 % alcohol beer. If you are on a sodium-restricted diet, canned tomato or vegetable juice should not be consumed more than once or twice a week. For a special occasion, order a spritzer (half soda water and half white wine). If you are drinking alcohol, try to limit your intake to a 150 ml (5 oz) glass of wine, a 45 ml (1 1/2 oz) serving of hard alcohol, or a beer.

Starter

Choose a green salad with raw vegetables, and ask for the dressing on the side. Choose a broth or potage, and ask if it is milk or cream-based. Choose whole-wheat bread without butter, and be careful not to eat too much of it. Avoid fat as much as possible. If you order a Caesar salad, ask for the dressing on the side.

Main course

Choose a dish that is low in fat. Look for the following key-words: steamed, grilled, poached, in its own juice, with tomato sauce, plain. When possible, choose restaurants where health-conscious food is served. Always ask for the sauce to be served on the side, and use it sparingly. If servings are big, do not feel obliged to finish your plate. If you have a sodium restriction, be careful with marinated and smoked food.

Pizza can be nourishing, but avoid pepperoni, anchovies, bacon and smoked meat. Instead, order a vegetable or seafood pizza. In fast-food restaurants the best choices are: a plain hamburger with lettuce and tomato, a grilled chicken sandwich, fajitas or a meat submarine without mayonnaise (roast beef, grilled chicken), or a grilled-vegetable panini.

Side dishes

Choose a baked or boiled potato, vegetables, steamed rice or plain pasta, rather than fries, vegetables in sauce or fried rice.

Dessert

Complete your meal with a light dessert: fresh fruit in a fruit cup or plain sorbet, flavored gelly, a milk-based dessert, frozen yogourt or angel food cake. Ask for 2% milk rather than cream for your coffee.

ADVICE FOR FOREIGN CUISINES

Chinese or Vietnamese cuisine

Beware of deep-fried food. Instead, order the dishes with vegetables and steamed rice. Avoid buffets because they tempt you to eat more. Many Chinese dishes are very salty; if possible, ask for the dish to be prepared with a lesser quality of salt and without MSG. Opt for dishes in which food is boiled, steam-cooked or lightly stir-fried in vegetable oil.

French cuisine

Hollandaise, béchamel made with cream, and béarnaise sauces must all be avoided. Instead, choose sauces based on wine (bordelaise), tomato (provençale) or milk (béchamel). Onion soup and dishes with melted cheese are also to be avoided.

Greek cuisine

Greek food is often high in fat. Choose a tzatziki (a yogourt-cucumber sauce), a salad, a kebab (brochette of lamb and grilled vegetables) and a baked tomato-based dish. Be careful of anything made with filo dough, for it will be high in fat.

Indian cuisine

Indian food is highly spiced and low in fat. The only food to avoid is ghee (clarified butter), which is used to cook vegetables. Salads and dishes with chicken, fish or lentils are all ideal choices.

Italian cuisine

Pasta is excellent for the health. As fresh pasta is prepared with eggs, calculate one egg per 150 g (1 cup) serving. However, avoid dishes with fatty meat, butter or cream. The following sauces are most recommended: marsala, mariana, primavera and wine-based. Breaded veal and chicken, such as parmigiana, must be avoided because they are high in fat. Eat bread without butter, or ask for margarine. For dessert, choose Italian ice cream (gelato).

Japanese cuisine

Japanese food is very salty but generally low in fat. Choose the vegetarian dishes and steamed rice. The beef and chicken dishes are also good choices. The dishes to avoid are those which are fried (tempura), salty soups (miso) and sauces. Sushi is a very good choice, but avoid those which contain fried ingredients.

Mexican cuisine

Mexican food is healthy and nourishing, for example, burritos (strips of beef and cheese with vegetables rolled into a corn-meal tortilla) and tacos (tortillas containing meat, red bean purée, lettuce, sour cream and guacamole) as well as spiced grilled meats, poultry and fish. Ceviche (fish marinated in lemon or lime juice) is an excellent choice. Avoid nachos (deep-fried tortillas with melted cheese and oil) and guacamole (avocado purée) because they are very high in fat. Request that the sour cream and cheese be served on the side.

Eastern European cuisine

Borsch (beet soup) with yogourt, cabbage rolls and pirogis (raviolis stuffed with potato and cottage cheese) are highly recommended.

MISCELLANEOUS ADVICE FOR RESTAURANT DINING
Buffets

All-you-can-eat buffets can be an excellent opportunity for trying new foods. However, it is important to choose items that are low in fat; avoid cold cuts and salads containing a great deal of mayonnaise or dressing. Learn to listen to your hunger to avoid overeating.

Seafood

Fried, fish *à la meunière* (floured and fried with butter and lemon), or in casseroles, or cream-based soups (clam chowder, for example) are to be avoided. Check to see if they are made with cream. Instead, choose dishes that are poached, grilled or cooked without added fat. If you want sauce, have it served on the side and use only a small quantity, or season your fish with lemon or lime juice.

Fondues

Fondues are to be avoided at restaurants. The oil used for beef fondue is not always the kind most recommended, and the bouillons in Chinese fondues are often high in salt. Go easy on the dipping sauce.

From the grill

Choose a filet mignon, flank or round steak, and limit your serving to 120 to 180 g (4 to 6 oz). If possible, ask for the meat to be cooked without fat, and that visible fat be removed before cooking; avoid eating chicken skin and gravy. Avoid fries; instead, order your meat with vegetables, a baked potato or rice, and a green salad.

Chapter 14 # Anticoagulant therapy and Vitamin K

DEFINITION

Anticoagulant therapy can be defined as the taking of certain medications such as warfarin or Sintrom, to prevent the formation of blood clots inside your heart or around your prosthetic cardiac valve, by slowing down your blood's coagulation.

ANTICOAGULANTS AND VITAMIN K

Vitamin K plays an essential role in the blood's coagulation. It promotes the formation of a clot when you are bleeding. However, anticoagulants and vitamin K work at odds with one another in the process of coagulation. A way must be found to use them without their canceling each other out. Vitamin K is principally found in certain green vegetables. You must certainly not remove these vegetables from your diet if you are in the habit of eating them. They may contain many other vitamins that are essential to health.

VITAMIN K AND DIET

A person being treated with anticoagulant medication must make sure that he or she has neither a deficiency nor an excess of Vitamin K. Their diet must contain a sufficient quantity of Vitamin K, and it must be ingested in a balanced and consistent way, because major fluctuations could prove dangerous.

You can ensure that your diet will not interfere with your anticoagulant medication by respecting the following indications:

- Know which foods are high in vitamin K (see list p.87).
- Eat only one vitamin K-rich food per day and stick to the recommended serving size. You are not obligated to eat one every day. However, it is important each week to consume the same quantity of foods high in vitamin K. For example: if you eat broccoli three times in one week, the week after, choose three other foods from the list of foods high in vitamin K (see below).
- Do not include foods high in vitamin K in your menu if you do not like them.
- Avoid drastic changes in your dietary habits (weight-reduction diet, becoming

vegetarian, adding a daily item in excess of your eating plan).

- Inform health care professionals of all major changes or any circumstances that might affect the stability of the INR (e.g.: travel, a personal loss, change of medicine, appearance of an illness).
- Alcool can be consumed only occasionally (1 or 2 /day).
- Avoid natural supplements that may interfere with your anticoagulant. Take supplements under medical supervision only.
- Vitamin K supplements or multivitamins containing vitamin K are to be avoided, and so are any other commercial nutritional formulas enriched with vitamin K.

Certain foods are higher in vitamin K than others. We suggest that you respect the quantities indicated. These are:

FOODS HIGH IN VITAMIN K

Foods	Maximum serving
Asparagus	250 ml (1 cup)
Swiss chard (raw)	125 ml (1/2 cup)
Broccoli	3 flowerets
Brussels sprouts	4
Green cabbage	250 ml (1 cup)
Raw spinach	250 ml (1 cup)
Boston lettuce	250 ml (2 cups)
Red lettuce	250 ml (1 cup)
Mung beans	125 ml (1/2 cup)

- You can choose only one of these foods per day and do not exceed the suggested serving size. If these vegetables are not ones you normally eat, you are not obligated to start eating them. As for green vegetables not on this list, you may eat them as you wish because they do not contain much vitamin K.
- Sushi made with algae should not be eaten as a main course, for it is very rich in vitamin K.
- Avoid collards and kale.
- Use fresh herbs as a seasoning only.

NATURAL AND VITAMIN SUPPLEMENTS

Over-the-counter vitamin supplements may interact with your medication. Considering their risk to the action of Coumadin (warfarin), the following are to be avoided:

- Vitamin E
- Folic acid
- Algae pills
- Ginseng
- Garlic pills
- Ginkgo
- Glucosamine, chondroitin
- Omega-3
- Coenzyme Q10
- Dong quai
- Red sage
- Millepertuis (Saint Johnswort)

Do not take other supplements except under strict medical supervision.

Chapter 15 Self-evaluation and self-instruction guide

This self-evaluation and self-instruction guide will help you evaluate how well-balanced your diet is. It will also help you analyse your eating habits in terms of the recommendations previously outlined, concerning dietary fats, cholesterol, concentrated sugar, fibre and salt. Moreover, it will outline the habits you need to acquire, and new dietary behavior to adopt.

But before you move into the action phase, it is important for you to be aware of your present eating habits. Begin by writing down everything you eat over the course of a day, for three days (two weekdays and one day over the weekend). This will help you visualize your personal eating habits and fill out the following exercise. We suggest that you fill it out with the person who usually prepares your meals and does the grocery-shopping.

Changing our eating habits cannot be done overnight. There is no miracle method. Of course patience and perseverance are necessary, but the results are worth it: a sense of encouragement and improvement in health. To make things easier, we suggest that you fill-out the charts at pages 90 to 94).

1. a) Put a check-mark in the blank next to "acquired habit", if the habit is already part of your daily life.

b) Check "habit to acquire" if the habit is not yet part of your daily life. This means it is a behavior you still need to adopt.

2. a) Among the "habit to acquire" boxes, choose the one that seems easiest to you. Select only one at a time and write in the box marked "starting date" the date when you will begin to change this habit. You can also combine two changes if one involves a reduction and the other an increase (less fat and more vegetables, for example).

b) In the "arrival date" box, write the date when you acquire this behavior. Then pass on to the next change to be made (habit to acquire).

The self-evaluation and self-instruction guide allows you to evaluate:

1. how well-balanced your diet is;

2. your consumption habits as far as saturated fats and cholesterol are concerned, as well concentrated sugar and alcohol, dietary fibre and salt.

DIETARY BALANCE

	Habit acquired	Habit to acquire	Starting date	Arrival date
Every day I consume:				
2 to 3 servings of milk and dairy products	☐	☐	_____	_____
6 to 8 servings of grain products	☐	☐	_____	_____
2 to 3 servings of meat, poultry, fish or alternative	☐	☐	_____	_____
7 to 10 servings of fruits and vegetables	☐	☐	_____	_____

N. B.: For serving sizes, consult *Eating Well with Canada's Food Guide*.

SOURCES OF SATURATED FAT AND CHOLESTEROL

These dietary changes particularly concern people with high cholesterol and those who want to base their diet on the recommendations of the Canadian Consensus Conference on Cholesterol.

	Habit acquired	Habit to acquire	Starting date	Arrival date
I skim the fat from soups and sauces cooled in the refrigerator.	☐	☐	_____	_____
I choose lean cuts of meat (e.g.: lean hamburger).	☐	☐	_____	_____
I trim all visible fat from meat before cooking it.	☐	☐	_____	_____
I trim the skin and fat from poultry before cooking it.	☐	☐	_____	_____
I use little or no fat for cooking.	☐	☐	_____	_____
I avoid fried foods.	☐	☐	_____	_____
I eat poultry at least twice a week.	☐	☐	_____	_____
I eat fish at least twice a week.	☐	☐	_____	_____
I limit my consumption of liver or other organ meats to once a week.	☐	☐	_____	_____

SOURCES OF SATURATED FAT AND CHOLESTEROL (suite)

	Habit acquired	Habit to acquire	Starting date	Arrival date
I eat a maximum of two egg yolks per week.	☐	☐	_____	_____
I limit my consumption of shrimp to four or five (medium-sized) per serving.	☐	☐	_____	_____
When I eat cold cuts, I choose products with reduced fat and salt, as indicated on the label.	☐	☐	_____	_____
I avoid eating frozen fries, even those without cholesterol.	☐	☐	_____	_____
I choose cheeses with less than 20% M.F.	☐	☐	_____	_____
I choose skim, 1 or 2% milk.	☐	☐	_____	_____
I make my milk-based desserts from skim, 1 or 2% milk.	☐	☐	_____	_____
I choose yogourt with 2% or less fat.	☐	☐	_____	_____
For cooking, I use yogourt or skim-milk cheese (e.g: white cheese, quark, etc.) to replace cream and sour cream.	☐	☐	_____	_____
For spreading, I use a soft margarine with less than 20% or 1.5 g of saturated fat per serving.	☐	☐	_____	_____
When I use fat for cooking, I mix half margarine and half monounsaturated fat (canola or olive oil) and limit the quantities I use.	☐	☐	_____	_____
For cooking, I replace butter, lard and shortening with margarine or recommended oils.	☐	☐	_____	_____
I read the labels on food in order to check the levels of saturated fats to be avoided: palm or palm kernel oil, coconut oil, hydrogenated oil.	☐	☐	_____	_____
I consume no more than 4 to 6 tsp. of fat per day.	☐	☐	_____	_____

SOURCES OF CONCENTRATED SUGAR AND ALCOHOL

These dietary changes primarily concern diabetics or those with high levels of triglycerides or who are obese, as well as anyone who wants to eat according to the recommendations of the Canadian Consensus Conference on Cholesterol.

	Habit acquired	Habit to acquire	Starting date	Arrival date
I replace regular soft drinks with dietetic soft drinks, or even better, with water or unsweetened fruit juices.	☐	☐	_____	_____
I replace alcoholic beverages with non-alcoholic beer or wine.	☐	☐	_____	_____
I choose unsweetened fruit juice instead of soft drinks or nectars.	☐	☐	_____	_____
I am gradually reducing the quantity of sugar, honey or other kinds of sugar, in my hot drinks, or use an artificial sweetener.	☐	☐	_____	_____
I replace refined breakfast cereals with whole-grain cereals with no added sugar.	☐	☐	_____	_____
I mix fruit into my cereal instead of sugar or honey.	☐	☐	_____	_____
I reserve cakes and pastries for special occasions; I make them myself with recommended fats (p. 42) and whole-wheat flour, reducing the quantity of sugar.	☐	☐	_____	_____
I avoid buying food products high in concentrated sugars (see p. 52).	☐	☐	_____	_____
Instead of icing, I use yogourt or fruit coulis.	☐	☐	_____	_____
I use pie filling without added sugar, and prepare the crust with margarine.	☐	☐	_____	_____
I appease my sweet-tooth with dried fruit or candy low in concentrated sugars.	☐	☐	_____	_____
I use plain cookies filled with light jam rather than cookies with cream fillings, chocolate or marshmallow.	☐	☐	_____	_____
I used fruits canned in their own juices and rinse them with cold water to remove sugar.	☐	☐	_____	_____

SOURCES OF DIETARY FIBRE

	Habit acquired	Habit to acquire	Starting date	Arrival date
I eat whole-grain cereals with a low sugar content (less than 5 g of sugar per serving) and which contain a minimum of 2 g of fibre per serving.	☐	☐	_____	_____
I increase my intake of fibre by eating baked goods made with whole grains.	☐	☐	_____	_____
I add oat bran to my recipes (e.g.: meatloaf, muffins).	☐	☐	_____	_____
I eat at least 3 to 5 pieces of fruit and 3 to 5 raw or cooked vegetables per day.	☐	☐	_____	_____
I eat one serving (3/4 to 1 cup) of cooked legumes at least once a week (e.g.: lentils, white or red kidney beans, chick peas, etc.).	☐	☐	_____	_____
I add legumes to soups, salads, and cooked dishes.	☐	☐	_____	_____
I eat the edible skin of fruit and vegetables.	☐	☐	_____	_____
I replace sugar with dried fruit and nuts in cereal and home-made desserts.	☐	☐	_____	_____

SOURCES OF SALT

	Habit acquired	Habit to acquire	Starting date	Arrival date
I replace broth concentrate (cubes, powder or liquid) with home-made broths, low in salt with fat removed, or concentrates low in fat and salt.	☐	☐	_____	_____
I eat home-made soups low in salt rather than soups from cans or packets.	☐	☐	_____	_____
I choose unsalted crackers.	☐	☐	_____	_____
I limit my intake of tomato or vegetable juice to 120 ml (1/2 cup) twice a week; if I want more, I mix the juice half-and-half with unsalted tomato juice.	☐	☐	_____	_____
I lightly salt my cooking and avoid using salt at the table.	☐	☐	_____	_____
For seasoning, I use fine herbs, powdered spices, home-made salad dressing, garlic, onions, black pepper and flavored peppers.	☐	☐	_____	_____

Chapter 16 Nutritional analysis

All the recipes in this book were analyzed with the Nutrisiq software. The data base for this software is the Canadian Nutrient file, 2005 version. The figures in the nutrition facts should be considered approximate due to the differences between one nutrition facts table and another, and also due to numerous factors that produce varied outcomes when a recipe is prepared.

To calculate the diabetic exchanges,

- We first determined the serving sizes for foods used in the recipes.
- We then identified the food groups whose quantities were sufficient for us to keep them as an exchange.

With the help of the *Guide d'alimentation pour la personne diabétique*, (available to order, in French only, by fax at 418 644-4574 or at communications@msss.gouv.qc.ca) we determined the quantity of protein, carbohydrates and lipids belonging to each food group.

- We determined the number of exchanges for each food group for each recipe in this manual.
- For each recipe, we have indicated the quantity of ingredients in both metric and imperial measures. Due to the slight differences between the two systems, it is better to choose one and use it for the entire recipe.
- The recipes made in the microwave were tested in a 650-watt oven. The cooking times are indicated for an oven of 650 to 700 watts. If the power of your oven is different, you should probably modify the cooking times. Check the owner's manual for your microwave oven. It if does not have a revolving platter, you should turn the dishes manually once or twice during cooking.
- The nutritional value of raw meats, poultry and fish was used in calculating the recipes. These foods lose some of their food value when they are cooked or served with sauce. As we mentioned before, it is important to remove fat from cooking liquid before eating it.
- In the recipes, the servings of meat, poultry and fish are 150 g (5 oz). These quantities are higher than the ones recommended in *Canada's Food Guide*. Cooking

causes a loss of volume estimated at 20 to 25%, that is, around 30 to 45 g (1 to 1 1/2 oz). The recommendation in *Canada's Food Guide* is 75 g cooked (2 1/4 oz), that is, an average acceptable quantity that is sufficient for the needs of a sedentary person. If you are sedentary, why not think about reducing the serving size of your meat, poultry or fish for your second meal of the day?

Now all you need to do is treat yourself to a delicious meal. The following chapters provide a wealth of tasty recipes to choose from. Enjoy!

PART 2
Recipes

99

Starters and appetizers

Lobster canapés

24 SERVINGS

NUTRITIONAL VALUE PER SERVING		
	Amount	% DV
Calories	40	
Fat	1.5 g	3%
Saturated	0 g	2%
+ Trans	0 g	
Polyunsaturated	1 g	
Omega-6	0.8 g	
Omega-3 (ALA)	0.1 g	
Omega-3 (EPA+DHA)	0 g	
Monounsaturated	0.5 g	
Cholesterol	6 mg	2%
Sodium	133 mg	6%
Potassium	43 mg	2%
Carbohydrate	5 g	2%
Dietary fibre	0.5 g	2%
Sugars	2 g	
Protein	2 g	
Vitamin A		2%
Vitamin C		11%
Calcium		2%
Iron 2%		
Vitamin D		1%
Vitamin E		3%

DIABETIC EXCHANGE
None

7.5 oz (225 g)	canned lobster or crab
4	chopped green onions
1	garlic clove, minced
3 tbsp. of each:	red, green and yellow peppers
1/4 cup (60 ml)	celery, finely chopped
1/3 cup (80 ml)	light mayonnaise
1/4 cup (60 ml)	plain fat-free yogourt
1 tsp.	lemon juice
1 tbsp.	chopped fresh oregano or 1/2 tsp. dried oregano
1/4 tsp.	salt
1 pinch	pepper
2 tbsp.	chopped parsley
12	mini-pitas

- Drain the lobster and coarsely chop. Add green onions, garlic, peppers and celery; mix well.
- In a small bowl, combine mayonnaise, yogourt, lemon juice and oregano.
- Combine the two mixtures. Add salt, pepper and parsley.
- With kitchen scissors, trim a thin border off the edges of the mini-pitas, and divide each in two horizontally. Arrange on a cookie sheet and dry in the oven at 350 °F (180 °C) for 10 minutes. Let them cool and spread with lobster salad. Garnish with fresh parsley sprigs. Serve.

Tomato aspic

8 SERVINGS

1 envelope	flavourless gelatine
1 envelope	low-calorie lemon gelatine (e.g. Jell-O Light)
1 cup (250 ml)	finely chopped celery
10	stuffed olives, rinsed in cold water and finely chopped
1/2 cup (125 ml)	small green onions, finely chopped
1 cup (250 ml)	boiling vegetable juice
1 1/4 cups (300 ml)	cold vegetable juice
1/4 cup (60 ml)	cold water

- Pour the envelope of flavourless gelatine in cold water and allow to swell. Set aside.
- Dissolve lemon gelatine in boiling vegetable juice. Stir well. Add the cold vegetable juice, stirring.
- Melt the gelatine in the microwave 20 seconds or by putting the dish in a saucepan with a few inches of boiling water. Add to tomato jelly. Stir and allow to cool.
- Add vegetables, pour all ingredients into an attractive mould, well-oiled and refrigerated ahead of time.
- Let set overnight. Unmould, decorate and serve.
- You can also pour the mixture into individual moulds. Unmould them onto lettuce leaves.

NUTRITIONAL VALUE PER SERVING

	Amount	% DV
Calories	35	
Fat	0.7 g	1%
Saturated	0 g	1%
+ Trans	0 g	
Polyunsaturated	0.2 g	
Omega-6	0.1 g	
Omega-3 (ALA)	0.1 g	
Omega-3 (EPA+DHA)	0 g	
Monounsaturated	0.5 g	
Cholesterol	0 mg	0%
Sodium	248 mg	11%
Potassium	196 mg	6%
Carbohydrate	5 g	2%
Dietary Fibre	1 g	4%
Sugars	5 g	
Protein	2 g	
Vitamin A		7%
Vitamin C		36%
Calcium		3%
Iron		5%
Vitamin D		0%
Vitamin E		4%

DIABETIC EXCHANGE

1 vegetables & fruits exchange

Dried tomato canapés

12 SERVINGS

NUTRITIONAL VALUE PER SERVING

	Amount	% DV
Calories	70	
Fat	1.5 g	3%
Saturated	0.5 g	3%
+ Trans	0 g	
Polyunsaturated		0.5 g
Omega-6	0.3 g	
Omega-3 (ALA)	0.1 g	
Omega-3 (EPA+DHA)	0 g	
Monounsaturated	0.5 g	
Cholesterol	2 mg	1%
Sodium	111 mg	5%
Potassium	103 mg	3%
Carbohydrate	11 g	4%
Dietary Fibre	1.5 g	6%
Sugars	5 g	
Protein	3 g	
Vitamin A		1%
Vitamin C		4%
Calcium		4%
Iron		6%
Vitamin D		0%
Vitamin E		1%

DIABETIC EXCHANGE

1/2 grain product exchange

8 slices	whole-wheat bread
3 tbsp.	chopped dried tomatoes
1/2 cup (125 ml)	home-made yogourt cheese (see recipe, p. 108)
1	garlic clove, finely chopped
1 tsp.	oregano

- Preheat oven to 350 °F (180 °C). Remove bread crusts and cut each slice into 6 little canapés. Place on a cookie sheet and toast in the oven for 12 to 15 minutes. Let cool and arrange in a cookie tin.
- Finely chop the dried tomatoes and add them to the cheese along with the garlic and oregano. Mix well, cover and refrigerate. Just before serving, spread the yogourt cheese mixture on each little piece of toasted bread. Garnish. Serve with before-dinner drinks.

Note The best way of cutting the bread into canapés is to use kitchen scissors. Both mixtures can be prepared 24 hours ahead of time.

Yogourt-fruit cup

8 SERVINGS

NUTRITIONAL VALUE PER SERVING

	Amount	% DV
Calories	165	
Fat	0.5 g	1%
Saturated	0 g	0%
+ Trans	0 g	
Polyunsaturated		0.5 g
Omega-6	0.2 g	
Omega-3 (ALA)	0.1 g	
Omega-3 (EPA+DHA)	0 g	
Monounsaturated	0 g	
Cholesterol	1 mg	1%
Sodium	37 mg	2%
Potassium	626 mg	18%
Carbohydrate	36 g	12%
Dietary Fibre	4.5 g	19%
Sugars	26 g	
Protein	4 g	
Vitamin A		13%
Vitamin C		166%
Calcium		10%
Iron		4%
Vitamin D		2%
Vitamin E		7%

DIABETIC EXCHANGE

2 1/2 vegetables & fruits exchanges

2	oranges
1	pink grapefruit
1	white grapefruit
1	red apple,
2	pears, ripe but firm
2	kiwifruits
1 cup (250 ml)	seedless red grapes
1 cup (250 ml)	seedless green grapes
1	cantaloupe, cut in half and seeded
1/2 cup (125 ml)	orange juice
2 tbsp.	lemon juice
1/4 cup (60 ml)	crème de cassis or Grand Marnier (optional)
1 cup (250 ml)	plain fat-free yogourt
2 tbsp.	low-calorie sweetener (Splenda)
1/2 tsp.	vanilla
1 tsp.	very fine orange zest

- Remove skin and pith (white inner skin) of the oranges and grapefruit, holding them over a bowl. Press fruits to extract the juice. Cut apple and pears, peel and slice kiwis. Cut the grapes in half. Using a small melon scoop, remove cantaloupe pulp, forming little balls. Combine orange juice, lemon juice and the juice from the the fruit. Add crème de cassis or Grand Marnier, if using. Sprinkle the syrup over the fruit. Mix gently. Refrigerate.
- Mix yogourt, sweetener and vanilla. Refrigerate.
- Just before serving, place the fruit in individual dishes or parfait glasses and pour the yogourt sauce over top. Garnish with orange zest.

Note This elegant starter replaces the traditional orange juice in a brunch.

Stuffed zucchini

8 SERVINGS

NUTRITIONAL VALUE PER SERVING

	Amount	% DV
Calories	65	
Fat	3 g	6%
Saturated	0.5 g	3%
+ Trans	0 g	
Polyunsaturated	1.5 g	
Omega-6	1.2 g	
Omega-3 (ALA)	0.2 g	
Omega-3 (EPA+DHA)	0 g	
Monounsaturated	1 g	
Cholesterol	0 mg	0%
Sodium	227 mg	10%
Potassium	406 mg	7%
Carbohydrate	9 g	3%
Dietary Fibre	2 g	9%
Sugars	3 g	
Protein	2 g	
Vitamin A		4%
Vitamin C		48%
Calcium		3%
Iron		7%
Vitamin D		0%
Vitamin E		9%

DIABETIC EXCHANGE

1 vegetables & fruits exchange

4	small zucchini
1/2 cup (125 ml)	finely minced onion
1	garlic clove, minced
1/3 cup (80 ml)	salad dressing, Italian dressing, Pink herb dressing or Tarragon dressing (see recipes, p. 228, 229, 227)
2 tbsp.	lemon juice

STUFFING:

1	red tomato
1	celery stick, finely chopped
3 tbsp.	red pepper, finely chopped
1 tbsp.	stuffed olives, rinsed in cold water and chopped
1	dried shallot, minced
1/2 tsp.	dry thyme or 1 tsp. fresh thyme
1/2 tsp.	paprika
1/4 tsp.	salt
	Pepper to taste
1 tbsp.	salad dressing (whichever one you chose above)

- Wash zucchini and remove ends. Cook in boiling water 5 minutes. The zucchini must still be crunchy. Rinse in cold water. Drain and cut in two lengthwise. With a spoon, remove and discard the seeds.
- Place zucchini in a covered dish.
- Combine the onion and garlic. Spread them over each zucchini half, and sprinkle with salad dressing and lemon juice. Cover and allow to marinate for at least 3 hours in the refrigerator.
- Prepare the filling. Blanch the tomato for several seconds. Plunge in cold water and peel.
- Remove seeds and juice, and chop the pulp.
- Combine with the other filling ingredients. Sprinkle with 1 tbsp. of salad dressing and mix.
- Remove and discard the garlic-onion mixture from the zucchini. Drain.
- Spread the filling in each zucchini half.
- Serve as an appetizer, on a lettuce leaf. Garnish with parsley sprigs.
- This dish also makes a welcome addition to a cold buffet.

Healthy pork paté

NUTRITIONAL VALUE PER 1 TBSP. SERVING		
	Amount	**% DV**
Calories	35	
Fat	2 g	4%
Saturated	0.5 g	4%
+ Trans	0 g	
Polyunsaturated	0.5 g	
Omega-6	0.4 g	
Omega-3 (ALA)	0 g	
Omega-3 (EPA+DHA)	0 g	
Monounsaturated	1 g	
Cholesterol	8 mg	3%
Sodium	43 mg	2%
Potassium	43 mg	2%
Carbohydrate	1 g	1%
Dietary Fibre	0 g	1%
Sugars	1 g	
Protein	3 g	
Vitamin A		1%
Vitamin C		1%
Calcium		1%
Iron		2%
Vitamin D		3%
Vitamin E		3%

DIABETIC EXCHANGE
None

1 lb (500 g)	lean minced pork*
1 cup (250 ml)	whole-wheat bread, crusts removed, chopped
1	onion, finely chopped
1	garlic clove, chopped
1 1/4 cup (300 ml)	1% milk
1/4 tsp.	Jamaican pepper
1/2 tsp.	savory
3/4 tsp.	salt
1 pinch	pepper
2 tbsp.	canola oil

- Mix all ingredients in a heavy cooking pot. Cover and simmer at very low heat, stirring from time to time, for 1 hour.
- To obtain a creamier texture, the cretons can be put through a mixer after cooking.
- Pour into ramekins and refrigerate.

* Chopped lean pork is a piece of raw pork from which the fat has been completely removed, and which has been ground by you, because commercial ground pork is never completely lean. With a knife, finely chop the piece of pork from which you have removed the fat, or put it through a meat grinder, or by small cubes in a food processor. This last method is the easiest and also applies to all other recipes using ground pork: meatloaf, meatballs, spaghetti sauce, etc. It is a little longer to prepare, but it is the only way of removing fat from the meat. What's more, it's delicious!

Stuffed pear halves

6 SERVINGS

NUTRITIONAL VALUE PER SERVING

	Amount	% DV
Calories	70	
Fat	0.5 g	1%
Saturated	0.1 g	1%
+ Trans	0 g	
Polyunsaturated	0.3 g	
Omega-6	0.1 g	
Omega-3 (ALA)	0.1 g	
Omega-3 (EPA+DHA)	0.1 g	
Monounsaturated	0.1 g	
Cholesterol	20 mg	7%
Sodium	42 mg	2%
Potassium	162 mg	5%
Carbohydrate	12 g	4%
Dietary Fibre	1.5 g	6%
Sugars	10 g	
Protein	4 g	
Vitamin A		1%
Vitamin C		4%
Calcium		5%
Iron		4%
Vitamin D		1%
Vitamin E		2%

DIABETIC EXCHANGE

1 meat & alternatives exchange
1/2 vegetables & fruits exchange

6	pear halves canned in their own juice, drained, or if sweetened, rinsed and patted dry.
1/2 cup (125 ml)	home-made yogourt cheese flavoured with chives (see recipe, p. 108)
1/2 cup (125 ml)	small shrimp, chopped crab, or crab-flavoured pollock
1/4 cup (60 ml)	celery, finely chopped

- Drain pears well on a piece of paper towel.
- During this time, soften the cheese with a fork and add shrimps or crab and celery.
- Place a scoop of the mixture in the centre of each pear half.
- Place each stuffed pear half on a lettuce leaf, on individual plates. Garnish with a sprig of parsley.

Home-made yogourt cheese

MAKES 2/3 CUP (160 ML)

NUTRITIONAL VALUE PER 1 TBSP. SERVING		
	Amount	% DV
Calories	30	
Fat	0 g	1%
Saturated	0 g	1%
+ Trans	0 g	
Polyunsaturated	0 g	
Omega-6	0 g	
Omega-3 (ALA)	0 g	
Omega-3 (EPA+DHA)	0 g	
Monounsaturated	0 g	
Cholesterol	1 mg	1%
Sodium	108 mg	5%
Potassium	132 mg	4%
Carbohydrate	4 g	2%
Dietary Fibre	0 g	1%
Sugars	4 g	
Protein	3 g	
Vitamin A		1%
Vitamin C		2%
Calcium		8%
Iron		1%
Vitamin D		3%
Vitamin E		1%

DIABETIC EXCHANGE
None

2 cups (500 ml)	plain yogourt
1/4 tsp.	salt
1/4 tsp.	pepper
2 tbsp.	finely-chopped chives

- If you are making the yogourt yourself, omit the flavourless gelatine from your recipe. If you are using the store-bought kind, carefully read the list of ingredients and choose a brand of fat-free yogourt that does not contain gelatine.
- Through a bag made out of a piece of cheesecloth suspended over a large dish, drain the yogourt without gelatine for 6 to 8 hours or overnight. Discard liquid and place contents of the bag in a bowl. Season with salt, pepper and chives. Mix well and refrigerate.
- This cheese is delicious on rusks or whole-wheat toast. It can also be seasoned with 1 tsp. onion and 1 tbsp. finely chopped red pepper.

Two-salmon mousse

6 SERVINGS

NUTRITIONAL VALUE PER SERVING

	Amount	% DV
Calories	190	
Fat	7.5 g	12%
Saturated	3 g	17%
+ Trans	0 g	
Polyunsaturated	1.5 g	
Omega-6	0.3 g	
Omega-3 (ALA)	0.1 g	
Omega-3 (EPA+DHA)	0.9 g	
Monounsaturated	2.5 g	
Cholesterol	43 mg	15%
Sodium	736 mg	31%
Potassium	333 mg	10%
Carbohydrate	5 g	2%
Dietary Fibre	0.5 g	2%
Sugars	1 g	
Protein	25 g	
Vitamin A		8%
Vitamin C		3%
Calcium		26%
Iron		8%
Vitamin D		127%
Vitamin E		13%

DIABETIC EXCHANGE

3 1/2 meat & alternatives exchanges

1 envelope	flavourless gelatine
1/2 cup (125 ml)	cold water
15.5 oz (435 g)	canned salmon, drained
1/4 lb (125 g)	smoked salmon
1 cup (250 ml)	ricotta
1	dried shallot, chopped fine
2 tbsp.	chopped fresh dill
1 tbsp.	chopped fresh basil
1 tbsp.	chopped fresh chives
2	egg whites
1/2 tsp.	salt
1/4 tsp.	pepper

- Let gelatine sit in cold water for 5 minutes. Melt it down in the microwave for 30 seconds at high intensity (level 10) or by putting the dish in a saucepan with a few inches of boiling water. Stir until gelatine is dissolved. Set aside.
- Remove bones from salmon, and finely chop the two kinds of salmon in the food processor. Transfer to a large bowl. Add ricotta, shallot, dill, basil, chives and melted gelatine. Beat egg whites until they form stiff peaks. Gently fold them into the mixture. Add salt and pepper.
- Pour into 6 little ramekins sprayed with no-stick vegetable cooking spray. Refrigerate for several hours until firm. Unmould onto a lettuce leaf and garnish with a sprig of fresh dill.

Lobster mousse

10 SERVINGS

NUTRITIONAL VALUE PER SERVING		
	Amount	% DV
Calories	120	
Fat	4.5 g	8%
Saturated	1 g	5%
+ Trans	0 g	
Polyunsaturated	2 g	
Omega-6	2 g	
Omega-3 (ALA)	0.2 g	
Omega-3 (EPA+DHA)	0 g	
Monounsaturated	1.5 g	
Cholesterol	23 mg	8%
Sodium	333 mg	14%
Potassium	257 mg	8%
Carbohydrate	7 g	3%
Dietary Fibre	0.5 g	2%
Sugars	4 g	
Protein	13 g	
Vitamin A		3%
Vitamin C		12%
Calcium		6%
Iron		4%
Vitamin D		1%
Vitamin E		6%

2	fresh 1 lb (500 g) lobsters (10 oz/300 g of meat)
1 cup (250 ml)	1% cottage cheese
1/2 cup (125 ml)	light mayonnaise
1/2 cup (125 ml)	plain fat-free yogourt
1/3 cup (80 ml)	chili sauce
2	dried shallots, chopped fine
5 tbsp.	chopped parsley
1/8 tsp.	pepper
2 tbsp.	lemon juice
2 envelopes	flavourless gelatine
1/2 cup (125 ml)	cold water
3	egg whites

- Extract the meat from the two lobsters and finely chop. Combine in a large bowl with cottage cheese, mayonnaise, yogourt, chili sauce, shallots, parsley, pepper and lemon juice. Soak gelatine in cold water for 3 minutes. Melt it in the microwave for 20 seconds at high intensity (10) or by putting the dish in a saucepan with a few inches of boiling water. Add gelatine to the first mixture.
- Beat egg whites until they form stiff peaks.
- Carefully fold egg whites into the mixture. Pour into 10 little ramekins sprayed with no-stick vegetable cooking spray.
- Refrigerate until firm. Unmould or serve in ramekins with whole-wheat crackers.

DIABETIC EXCHANGE
1 meat & alternatives exchange
1/2 oils & fats exchange

111
Soups

Home-made beef broth

7 SERVINGS

(MICROWAVE OR TRADITIONAL METHOD)

NUTRITIONAL VALUE PER SERVING		
	Amount	% DV
Calories	25	
Fat	1 g	1%
Saturated	0 g	1%
+ Trans	0 g	
Polyunsaturated	0 g	
Omega-6	0.1 g	
Omega-3 (ALA)	0 g	
Omega-3 (EPA+DHA)	0 g	
Monounsaturated	0 g	
Cholesterol	0 mg	0%
Sodium	75 mg	3%
Potassium	209 mg	6%
Carbohydrate	3 g	2%
Dietary Fibre	0.5 g	0%
Sugars	1 g	
Protein	1 g	
Vitamin A		22%
Vitamin C		9%
Calcium		3%
Iron		4%
Vitamin D		0%
Vitamin E		3%

DIABETIC EXCHANGE
None

1	big soup bone
10 cups (2.5 litres)	boiling water
3	carrots cut in rounds
2	half-stalks of celery with leaves
1	onion cut in two
1	whole leek, well washed and cut into 1 inch (2.5 cm) sections
	Pepper to taste
1	bay leaf
1/2 tsp.	savory
1/4 tsp.	thyme

Microwave method:

- Broths can be made much more quickly in the microwave than on the stove-top, and are just as tasty and nutritious. They are less fatty and salty than commercial broths.
- Place all ingredients in a 20-cup (5-litre) microwave-safe receptacle. Cover and cook at high intensity (10) for 15 minutes. Reduce heat to medium intensity (7) and continue cooking for 1 1/2 hours.
- Strain the broth, thoroughly cool in the refrigerator, and skim the fat off, that is, remove and discard the thin layer of fat congealed at the surface of the liquid.

Stove-top method:

- With this cooking method, it is preferable to use cold water. Place all ingredients in a large stew pot. Slowly bring to a boil and let simmer for at least 3 hours.
- Strain the broth, let cool, and skim the fat off.

Note This broth freezes well and can be kept for up to 3 months in the freezer.

Home-made chicken broth

ABOUT 10 SERVINGS

(MICROWAVE OR TRADITIONAL METHOD)

	NUTRITIONAL VALUE PER SERVING		

	Amount	% DV
Calories	25	
Fat	1 g	1%
Saturated	0 g	1%
+ Trans	0 g	
Polyunsaturated	0 g	
Omega-6	0.1 g	
Omega-3 (ALA)	0 g	
Omega-3 (EPA+DHA)	0 g	
Monounsaturated	0 g	
Cholesterol	0 mg	0%
Sodium	75 mg	3%
Potassium	209 mg	6%
Carbohydrate	3 g	2%
Dietary Fibre	0.5 g	0%
Sugars	1 g	
Protein	1 g	
Vitamin A		22%
Vitamin C		9%
Calcium		3%
Iron		4%
Vitamin D		0%
Vitamin E		3%

DIABETIC EXCHANGE
None

1	raw or cooked poultry carcass
10 cups (2.5 litres)	boiling water
3	carrots cut into rounds
1	onion cut in pieces
2	half-stalks of celery with leaves
	Pepper to taste
1	bay leaf
1/2 tsp.	tarragon
1/4 tsp.	chervil

Microwave method:

- Place all ingredients in a 20-cup (5-litre) microwave-safe receptacle. Cover and boil at high intensity (10) for 45 minutes. Strain broth, allow to completely cool in the refrigerator and skim off the layer of fat that has formed on the surface.

Stove-top method:

- Replace boiling water from the preceding recipe with 2.5 litres (10 cups) cold water. Place all ingredients in a large soup pot. Slowly bring to a boil and let simmer for 2 hours.
- Strain broth, let cool, then skim off the fat.

Note Some of the broth can be frozen in ice-cube trays (certain recipes, such as sauces, require only a small quantity of broth). When the cubes are frozen, transfer into a sealable plastic bag. Both the beef and chicken broth freeze very well, and can be kept up to 3 months in the freezer.

Cream of zucchini soup

8 SERVINGS

2 cups (500 ml)	diced potatoes
2 cups (500 ml)	well-washed, unpeeled zucchini, diced
1	finely chopped onion
1	finely chopped leek
6 cups (1.5 litre)	hot home-made chicken broth (see recipe, p. 113) or a fat-free, salt-free commercial brand
1 cup (250 ml)	1% milk
1/2 tsp.	salt
	Pepper to taste
	Parsley to garnish

- Cook vegetables in a small quantity of water over medium heat. Put through the blender. Add to hot chicken broth. Season. Add milk.
- Just before serving, sprinkle each plate of soup with finely chopped parsley, or serve with a spoonful of plain yogourt in the centre. Delicious!

NUTRITIONAL VALUE PER SERVING

	Amount	% DV
Calories	80	
Fat	1 g	1%
Saturated	0.5 g	2%
+ Trans	0 g	
Polyunsaturated	0 g	
Omega-6	0 g	
Omega-3 (ALA)	0 g	
Omega-3 (EPA+DHA)	0 g	
Monounsaturated	0 g	
Cholesterol	2 mg	1%
Sodium	233 mg	10%
Potassium	518 mg	15%
Carbohydrate	14 g	5%
Dietary Fibre	1.5 g	7%
Sugars	2 g	
Protein	5 g	
Vitamin A		4%
Vitamin C		30%
Calcium		8%
Iron		9%
Vitamin D		7%
Vitamin E		2%

DIABETIC EXCHANGE

1/2 grain product exchange
1 vegetables & fruits exchange

Creamy autumn vegetable soup

8 SERVINGS

NUTRITIONAL VALUE PER SERVING

	Amount	% DV
Calories	110	
Fat	3 g	5%
Saturated	1 g	4%
+ Trans	0 g	
Polyunsaturated	0.5 g	
Omega-6	0.2 g	
Omega-3 (ALA)	0 g	
Omega-3 (EPA+DHA)	0 g	
Monounsaturated	1.5 g	
Cholesterol	3 mg	1%
Sodium	395 mg	17%
Potassium	666 mg	20%
Carbohydrate	17 g	6%
Dietary Fibre	2 g	9%
Sugars	3 g	
Protein	6 g	
Vitamin A		33%
Vitamin C		25%
Calcium		13%
Iron		9%
Vitamin D		13%
Vitamin E		11%

DIABETIC EXCHANGE

1/2 grain product exchange
1/2 oils & fats exchange
1/2 vegetables & fruits exchange

1 tbsp.	olive oil
1	chopped onion
1/2 cup (125 ml)	chopped celery
4 cups (1 litre)	cubed pumpkin
2	potatoes cut in cubes
2	carrots cut in rounds
4 cups (1 litre)	home-made chicken broth (see recipe p. 113), or fat-free, salt-free commercial brand
2 cups (500 ml)	1% milk
1/2 tsp.	finely ground coriander seeds
1/2 tsp.	sage
1 tsp.	salt
	Pepper to taste

- Heat oil in a non-stick saucepan. Add onion and celery. Soften for five minutes without letting them brown. Add pumpkin, potatoes, carrots and chicken broth. Bring to a rolling boil. Reduce heat and simmer 30 minutes, or until pumpkin becomes transparent.
- Mix in the blender or food processor. Pour back into the saucepan. Add milk, coriander and sage, salt and pepper.
- Avoid letting it boil again. Serve garnished with parsley sprigs.

Creamy watercress soup

6 SERVINGS

2 tbsp.	olive oil
1	leek (both white and green parts, sliced)
1	chopped onion
1 cup (250 ml)	potato, diced
1 bunch	watercress, washed with stems removed
5 cups (1.25 litre)	home-made chicken broth (see recipe p. 113), or
	fat-free salt-free commercial brand
1 cup (250 ml)	1% milk
1/2 tsp.	salt
	Pepper to taste

- Heat oil in a saucepan. Add leek and onion. Soften over medium heat for 5 minutes. Add potato, watercress and chicken broth. Allow to simmer until the potatoes are cooked.
- Mix in blender or food processor. Return to saucepan. Add milk and seasonings.
- Serve hot garnished with small toasted croutons.

Yellow bean soup

5 SERVINGS

2 cups (500 ml)	fresh yellow wax beans
1/2 cup (125 ml)	diced celery
1	minced onion
1 tbsp.	olive oil
1 tbsp.	flour
4 cups (1litre)	1% milk
1/2 tsp.	salt
	Pepper to taste
1 pinch	sage

- Wash the beans and snap the ends off. Cut into 1 inch (2.5 cm) pieces. Cook with celery and onion in boiling water until tender.
- Drain and set aside.
- Make a roux with the oil and flour. Add the skimmed milk and gently bring mixture to the boiling point, without letting it boil. Add vegetables and seasonings.

NUTRITIONAL VALUE PER SERVING

	Amount	% DV
Calories	160	
Fat	5 g	8%
Saturated	2 g	10%
+ Trans	0.1 g	
Polyunsaturated	0.5 g	
Omega-6	0.4 g	
Omega-3 (ALA)	0.1 g	
Omega-3 (EPA+DHA)	0 g	
Monounsaturated	2.5 g	
Cholesterol	9 mg	3%
Sodium	372 mg	16%
Potassium	550 mg	16%
Carbohydrate	19 g	7%
Dietary Fibre	2.5 g	10%
Sugars	3 g	
Protein	10 g	
Vitamin A		15%
Vitamin C		21%
Calcium		30%
Iron		6%
Vitamin D		42%
Vitamin E		7%

DIABETIC EXCHANGE

1 vegetables & fruits exchange
1/2 milk & alternatives exchange
1/2 oils & fats exchange

French onion soup

6 SERVINGS

1 tbsp.	olive oil
2 cups (500 ml)	sliced onions
1/2 tsp.	mustard powder
5 cups (1.25 litre)	home-made beef broth (see recipe, p. 112) or
	fat-free salt-free commercial broth
1/2 tsp.	marjoram
1/2 tsp.	salt
	Pinch of pepper
1/3 cup (80 ml)	light Emmenthal cheese (15% M.F.)
6	toasted slices of baguette, 3/4 inch (2 cm) thick

- In a large non-stick saucepan, heat oil. Add onion and mustard. Cook at low heat for 15 minutes, stirring often. Add broth, bring to a boil. Simmer, partly covered, for 15 minutes. Season.
- Pour into 6 oven-proof bowls, cover each with a slice of toasted baguette. Sprinkle the cheese over the 6 slices of bread. Put under the broiler. Serve immediately.

NUTRITIONAL VALUE PER SERVING

	Amount	% DV
Calories	145	
Fat	5 g	8%
Saturated	1.5 g	7%
+ Trans	0 g	
Polyunsaturated	0.5 g	
Omega-6	0.5 g	
Omega-3 (ALA)	0.1 g	
Omega-3 (EPA+DHA)	0 g	
Monounsaturated	2.5 g	
Cholesterol	5 mg	2%
Sodium	446 mg	19%
Potassium	320 mg	10%
Carbohydrate	18 g	7%
Dietary Fibre	2.5 g	11%
Sugars	7g	
Protein	8 g	
Vitamin A		1%
Vitamin C		6%
Calcium		9%
Iron		13%
Vitamin D		0%
Vitamin E		5%

DIABETIC EXCHANGE

1/2 vegetables & fruits exchange
1/2 grain product exchange
1/2 oils & fats exchange

Barley vegetable soup

8 SERVINGS

<table>
<tr><td>NUTRITIONAL VALUE
PER SERVING</td><td></td><td></td></tr>
<tr><td></td><td>Amount</td><td>% DV</td></tr>
<tr><td>Calories</td><td>90</td><td></td></tr>
<tr><td>Fat</td><td>0 g</td><td>1%</td></tr>
<tr><td>Saturated</td><td>0 g</td><td>1%</td></tr>
<tr><td>+ Trans</td><td>0 g</td><td></td></tr>
<tr><td>Polyunsaturated</td><td>0 g</td><td></td></tr>
<tr><td>Omega-6</td><td>0.1 g</td><td></td></tr>
<tr><td>Omega-3 (ALA)</td><td>0 g</td><td></td></tr>
<tr><td>Omega-3 (EPA+DHA)</td><td>0 g</td><td></td></tr>
<tr><td>Monounsaturated</td><td>0 g</td><td></td></tr>
<tr><td>Cholesterol</td><td>0 mg</td><td>0%</td></tr>
<tr><td>Sodium</td><td>537 mg</td><td>23%</td></tr>
<tr><td>Potassium</td><td>625 mg</td><td>18%</td></tr>
<tr><td>Carbohydrate</td><td>18 g</td><td>6%</td></tr>
<tr><td>Dietary Fibre</td><td>3 g</td><td>13%</td></tr>
<tr><td>Sugars</td><td>5 g</td><td></td></tr>
<tr><td>Protein</td><td>6 g</td><td></td></tr>
<tr><td>Vitamin A</td><td></td><td>12%</td></tr>
<tr><td>Vitamin C</td><td></td><td>39%</td></tr>
<tr><td>Calcium</td><td></td><td>8%</td></tr>
<tr><td>Iron</td><td></td><td>17%</td></tr>
<tr><td>Vitamin D</td><td></td><td>0%</td></tr>
<tr><td>Vitamin E</td><td></td><td>13%</td></tr>
</table>

DIABETIC EXCHANGE

2 vegetables & fruits exchanges

8 cups (2 litres)	home-made beef broth (see recipe, p. 112) or fat-free salt-free commercial broth
1 cup (250 ml)	chopped leek (both green and white parts)
1 cup (250 ml)	diced carrots
1 cup (250 ml)	diced celery
1 cup (250 ml)	diced parsnips
1/2 cup (125 ml)	diced turnip
1/4 cup (60 ml)	pearl barley
1/4 tsp.	oregano
1/2 tsp.	rosemary
1/4 tsp.	savory
1 tsp.	salt
	Pepper to taste
28 oz (796 ml)	diced canned tomatoes

- In a large saucepan, bring the beef broth to a boil. Add vegetables, barley and all seasonings. Simmer for 1 hour. Add tomatoes and cook for another 30 minutes. Serve.

Fresh tomato instant soup

4 SERVINGS

NUTRITIONAL VALUE PER SERVING

	Amount	% DV
Calories	105	
Fat	4 g	7%
Saturated	0.5 g	3%
+ Trans	0 g	
Polyunsaturated	0.5 g	
Omega-6	0.5 g	
Omega-3 (ALA)	0.1 g	
Omega-3 (EPA+DHA)	0 g	
Monounsaturated	2.5 g	
Cholesterol	0 mg	0%
Sodium	365 mg	16%
Potassium	624 mg	18%
Carbohydrate	16 g	6%
Dietary Fibre	3 g	13%
Sugars	3 g	
Protein	4 g	
Vitamin A		11%
Vitamin C		104%
Calcium		5%
Iron		12%
Vitamin D		0%
Vitamin E		14%

DIABETIC EXCHANGE

2 vegetables & fruits exchanges
1 oils & fats exchange

1 tbsp.	olive oil
1	onion finely chopped
1	dried shallot, finely minced
1/2	red pepper, finely chopped
2 cups (500 ml)	home-made chicken broth (see recipe, p. 113) or fat-free salt-free commercial broth
8	fresh Italian tomatoes
1/2 cup (125 ml)	chopped celery
1/4 cup (60 ml)	chopped parsley
1 tbsp.	fresh chopped basil
1/4 cup (60 ml)	finely minced chives
1/2 tsp.	salt
	Pepper to taste

- Blanch the tomatoes for 2 minutes. Cool in cold water.
- Peel and cut in cubes.
- In a large non-stick saucepan, heat the oil at low heat. Add onion, shallot and red pepper.
- Cook for 10 minutes without letting vegetables stick to the pan. Add broth, bring to a boil. Add tomatoes, celery, parsley, basil and chives. Let simmer for 10 minutes. Add salt and pepper. Serve.

Comforting pea soup

8 SERVINGS

NUTRITIONAL VALUE PER SERVING		
	Amount	% DV
Calories	260	
Fat	4 g	7%
Saturated	0.5 g	3%
+ Trans	0 g	
Polyunsaturated	1 g	
Omega-6	0.7 g	
Omega-3 (ALA)	0.1 g	
Omega-3 (EPA+DHA)	0 g	
Monounsaturated	2.5 g	
Cholesterol	0 mg	0%
Sodium	327 mg	14%
Potassium	726 mg	21%
Carbohydrate	42 g	14%
Dietary Fibre	5.5 g	22%
Sugars	7 g	
Protein	16 g	
Vitamin A		11%
Vitamin C		7%
Calcium		6%
Iron		22%
Vitamin D		0%
Vitamin E		7%

DIABETIC EXCHANGE
1 grain product exchange
1 oils & fats exchange
1 vegetables & fruits exchange

1 lb (500 g)	dry peas
8 cups (2 litres)	hot water
1 tsp.	salt
	Pepper to taste
1	large chopped onion
3/4 cup (180 ml)	diced celery
1 cup (250 ml)	diced carrots
2 tbsp.	olive oil
2 tsp.	savory

- Wash peas thoroughly and soak overnight. Drain. In a large saucepan mix peas, hot water, salt, pepper and onion. Simmer 1 hour.
- Add celery, carrots, oil and savory.
- Cook until all vegetables are tender.

Note Made without salt lard, and therefore without cholesterol, this delicious pea soup, served with a piece of whole-wheat bread, makes a nutritious meal in itself.

Cream of vegetable soup

10 SERVINGS

(MICROWAVE OR TRADITIONAL METHOD)

NUTRITIONAL VALUE PER SERVING

	Amount	% DV
Calories	110	
Fat	3 g	5%
Saturated	0.5 g	4%
+ Trans	0 g	
Polyunsaturated	1 g	
Omega-6	1 g	
Omega-3 (ALA)	0 g	
Omega-3 (EPA+DHA)	0 g	
Monounsaturated	1.5 g	
Cholesterol	2 mg	1%
Sodium	358 mg	15%
Potassium	609 mg	18%
Carbohydrate	16 g	6%
Dietary Fibre	2.5 g	10%
Sugars	3 g	
Protein	5 g	
Vitamin A		27%
Vitamin C		25%
Calcium		8%
Iron		9%
Vitamin D		6%
Vitamin E		9%

DIABETIC EXCHANGE

1/2 grain product exchange
1 vegetables & fruits exchange

2 tbsp.	olive oil
1	chopped onion
5	grated carrots
4	potatoes, cubed
1/2	grated turnip
3	sliced celery stalks
1	bay leaf
1 tsp.	*herbes de Provence* (see recipe, p. 259)
1 pinch	thyme
1 tsp.	salt
	Pepper and paprika to taste
8 cups (2 litres)	chilled home-made chicken broth (see recipe p. 113) or no-fat no-salt commercial broth
1 cup (250 ml)	1% milk

Microwave method:

- Heat oil in a 20-cup (5-litre) microwave-safe container. Add onion. Cook 3 minutes at high intensity (10). Add remaining ingredients except milk. Cook at high (10) for 15 minutes, then at medium (7) for 30 minutes. Mix vegetables in the blender or food processor. Combine with broth. Add milk, correct seasoning. Serve garnished with chopped fresh parsley or a few croutons.

Traditional method:

- Heat oil in a non-stick saucepan. Add onion and celery. Soften for 5 minutes without browning. Add remaining ingredients except milk. Bring to a boil, simmer 30 minutes. Remove bay leaf.
- Mix all ingredients in the blender or food processor. Return to saucepan. Add milk, correct seasoning.
- Serve garnished with parsley or croutons.

Note This creamy soup freezes well. Store in a container with a tightly-fitting lid, filling only three-quarters full. When ready to use, thaw in the refrigerator or the microwave.

Quick chicken soup

6 SERVINGS

5 cups (1.25 litre)	home-made chicken broth (see recipe p. 113), or no-fat no-salt commercial broth
1 ½ cups (375 ml)	grated vegetables: carrots, turnips, broccoli stems, etc.
2	celery stalks sliced thin
1 cup (250 ml)	leek, both white and green, chopped
½ cup (125 ml)	small soup pasta
⅔ cup (160 ml)	leftover cooked chicken, cut in cubes
½ tsp.	salt
	Pepper to taste

- In a large saucepan, bring the chicken broth to a boil. Add all vegetables. Boil for 5 minutes. Add pasta and continue cooking for 7 to 8 minutes, or until pasta is cooked.
- Add chicken, salt and pepper
- Return to a boil. Serve.

NUTRITIONAL VALUE PER SERVING

	Amount	% DV
Calories	95	
Fat	1 g	2%
Saturated	0 g	2%
+ Trans	0 g	
Polyunsaturated	0.5 g	
Omega-6	0.2 g	
Omega-3 (ALA)	0 g	
Omega-3 (EPA+DHA)	0 g	
Monounsaturated	0.5 g	
Cholesterol	12 mg	4%
Sodium	300 mg	13%
Potassium	373 mg	11%
Carbohydrate	13 g	5%
Dietary Fibre	1.5 g	7%
Sugars	2 g	
Protein	9 g	
Vitamin A		8%
Vitamin C		22%
Calcium		5%
Iron		12%
Vitamin D		1%
Vitamin E		4%

DIABETIC EXCHANGE

1 vegetables & fruits exchange
1 meat & alternatives exchange

125
Pasta and Rice

Fettuccine primavera

4 SERVINGS

NUTRITIONAL VALUE PER SERVING

	Amount	% DV
Calories	270	
Fat	2 g	4%
Saturated	0.5 g	2%
+ Trans	0 g	
Polyunsaturated	0.5 g	
Omega-6	0.5 g	
Omega-3 (ALA)	0.1 g	
Omega-3 (EPA+DHA)	0 g	
Monounsaturated	1 g	
Cholesterol	0 mg	0%
Sodium	317 mg	14%
Potassium	280 mg	8%
Carbohydrate	53 g	18%
Dietary Fibre	2.5 g	11%
Sugars	4 g	
Protein	9 g	
Vitamin A		4%
Vitamin C		73%
Calcium		3%
Iron		20%
Vitamin D		4%
Vitamin E		7%

DIABETIC EXCHANGE

1 grain product exchange
1 vegetables & fruits exchange

1 tsp.	olive oil
1	finely chopped large onion
1	garlic clove, minced
1/2 cup (125 ml)	finely chopped celery
1/2 cup (125 ml)	chopped red pepper
1/2 cup (125 ml)	chopped mushrooms
2 tsp.	lemon juice
1/2 tsp.	salt
	Pepper to taste
1/4 tsp.	oregano
1/2 lb (250 g)	fettuccine
1 tbsp.	chopped parsley

- Heat oil at medium heat in a heavy non-stick frying pan. Add onion, garlic, celery, pepper and mushrooms.
- Cook stirring for 5 minutes.
- Sprinkle with lemon juice and add seasoning. Cook the pasta in boiling water until it is "al dente". Drain. Add vegetable mixture and sprinkle with parsley. Serve very hot.

Citrus pilaf

6 SERVINGS

	Amount	% DV
NUTRITIONAL VALUE PER SERVING		
Calories	285	
Fat	8 g	13%
Saturated	1 g	5%
+ Trans	0 g	
Polyunsaturated	1 g	
Omega-6	1.1 g	
Omega-3 (ALA)	0.1 g	
Omega-3 (EPA+DHA)	0 g	
Monounsaturated	5.5 g	
Cholesterol	0 mg	0%
Sodium	234 mg	10%
Potassium	296 mg	9%
Carbohydrate	47 g	16%
Dietary Fibre	1 g	5%
Sugars	2 g	
Protein	7 g	
Vitamin A		1%
Vitamin C		23%
Calcium		5%
Iron		10%
Vitamin D		0%
Vitamin E		38%

DIABETIC EXCHANGE

2 1/2 grain product exchanges

2 tbsp.	olive oil
1	finely chopped onion
1	dried shallot, finely chopped
1/4 cup (60 ml)	flaked almonds
1 tsp.	orange zest
1/2 tsp.	lemon zest
1 tsp.	curry powder
1 1/2 cup (375 ml)	long-grain rice
1/4 cup (60 ml)	fresh orange juice
1/4 cup (60 ml)	fresh lemon juice
2 1/2 cups (625 ml)	home-made chicken broth (see recipe, p. 113) or no-fat no-salt commercial broth
1/2 tsp.	salt
2 tsp.	freshly chopped parsley

- Heat oil in a saucepan. Cook onion and shallot until tender but without letting them brown. Add almonds, orange and lemon zest, and curry. Mix well.
- Stirring, add rice, orange and lemon juice, and hot chicken broth. Reduce heat to low and cook 20 minutes, until all the liquid is absorbed. Add salt and pepper, sprinkle with parsley.

Curried rice

6 SERVINGS

2 cups (500 ml)	water
1 cup (250 ml)	long grain rice
½ tsp.	salt
1 tbsp.	olive oil
½ cup (125 ml)	finely chopped celery
2	small chopped green onions
1 tsp.	curry
½ tsp.	cumin

- Rinse rice in cold water to remove excess starch. Bring water to a boil in a saucepan with a tightly-fitting lid.
- Add rice and salt. Cover and cook at low heat for 15 minutes without lifting the lid. Meanwhile, heat oil in a non-stick frying pan, add celery and green onion, and cook until golden.
- Mix with rice, curry and cumin. Delicious with brochettes or any other lamb dish.

NUTRITIONAL VALUE PER SERVING

	Amount	% DV
Calories	140	
Fat	2.5 g	5%
Saturated	0.5 g	3%
+ Trans	0 g	
Polyunsaturated	1 g	
Omega-6	0.8 g	
Omega-3 (ALA)	0.1 g	
Omega-3 (EPA+DHA)	0 g	
Monounsaturated	1 g	
Cholesterol	0 mg	0%
Sodium	209 mg	9%
Potassium	79 mg	3%
Carbohydrate	27 g	9%
Dietary Fibre	0.5 g	3%
Sugars	1 g	
Protein	3 g	
Vitamin A		1%
Vitamin C		2%
Calcium		2%
Iron		4%
Vitamin D		0%
Vitamin E		6%

DIABETIC EXCHANGE

1 grain product exchange
½ oils & fats exchange

Vegetable rice

6 SERVINGS

(MICROWAVE METHOD)

1 cup (250 ml)	long-grain rice
2 cups (500 ml)	home-made chicken broth (see recipe p. 113) or fat-free, salt-free commercial brand
¹/2 tsp.	salt
1 tbsp.	olive oil
¹/2 cup (125 ml)	finely chopped mushrooms
4	chopped small green onions (both white and green parts)
¹/4 cup (60 ml)	chopped green pepper
¹/4 cup (60 ml)	chopped red pepper
1	finely diced tomato
	Chopped parsley, to taste

- Rinse rice in cold water to remove excess starch. Drain well.
- In an 8-cup (2-litre) microwave-safe receptacle, heat chicken broth, salt and oil, 5 minutes at high intensity (10) or until it boils.
- Add rice, stir, and cover. Cook 14 to 16 minutes at medium intensity (7).
- Let sit for 5 minutes. Keep covered so the rice will stay warm.
- While rice is cooking, prepare all vegetables except the tomato, then cook 4 minutes at high intensity (10) with 2 tbsp. water in a 4-cup (1-litre) container. Drain and mix with warm rice.
- Add diced tomato to mixture and stir gently.
- Sprinkle with a bit of chopped parsley. Serve hot.

Note Vegetables may be varied according to season.

Rice ring with fine herbs

6 SERVINGS

NUTRITIONAL VALUE PER SERVING

	Amount	% DV
Calories	145	
Fat	3 g	4%
Saturated	0.5 g	2%
+ Trans	0 g	
Polyunsaturated	0.5 g	
Omega-6	0.3 g	
Omega-3 (ALA)	0 g	
Omega-3 (EPA+DHA)	0 g	
Monounsaturated	2 g	
Cholesterol	0 mg	0%
Sodium	210 mg	9%
Potassium	90 mg	3%
Carbohydrate	27 g	9%
Dietary Fibre	0.5 g	3%
Sugars	0 g	
Protein	3 g	
Vitamin A		1%
Vitamin C		4%
Calcium		2%
Iron		4%
Vitamin D		0%
Vitamin E		5%

DIABETIC EXCHANGE

1 ½ grain product exchange

2 ¼ cups (560 ml)	water
1 tbsp.	olive oil
½ tsp.	salt
1 cup (250 ml)	rice
½ cup (125 ml)	finely diced celery
3	finely chopped green onions
½ tsp.	chopped fresh basil
½ tsp.	chopped fresh rosemary
½ tsp.	chopped fresh oregano

- Bring water, oil and salt to a boil. Add rice and reduce heat to medium-low. Cover and allow to simmer for 20 minutes, or until water is absorbed.
- Remove from heat, add celery, green onion and fine herbs. Mix well.
- Spray a 4-cup (1-litre) ring-shaped jelly mould with non-stick vegetable spray. Press the rice mixture into it, using the back of a spoon.
- This mixture can be made the day before and stored in the refrigerator. Just before serving, unmould rice onto a big platter and reheat in the microwave at medium intensity (7) for 12 to 15 minutes.

131

Vegetables

Vegetable brochettes

4 SERVINGS

(COOKED ON A BARBECUE)

1	small zucchini cut in 1 inch (2.5 cm) slices	
8	pearl onions	
1	red pepper cut in squares	
8	mushrooms caps	
8	cherry tomatoes or 2 large tomatoes quartered	

MARINADE:

1/2 cup (125 ml)	olive oil
1 tbsp.	lemon juice
2 tbsp.	white wine vinegar
2 tsp.	Dijon mustard
1 tsp.	basil
1/2 tsp.	thyme
1/2 tsp.	oregano
2	garlic cloves, chopped

- Blanch zucchini, onions, pepper and mushrooms for 5 minutes.
- Put all vegetables into a big salad bowl.
- Mix together marinade ingredients and pour over vegetables. Let marinate in a cool place for 2 hours.
- Drain vegetables and conserve marinade. Assemble the brochettes, alternating the different kinds of vegetables.
- Barbecue brochettes at approximately 6 inches (15 cm) from the heat source.
- Cook for approximately 10 minutes at low heat, turning and basting with marinade 2 or 3 times while cooking.

Note Vegetable brochettes make a perfect accompaniment for barbecued steaks or chops. If you don't use the marinade for cooking, you reduce your fat intake by 5 g.

NUTRITIONAL VALUE PER SERVING (1 BROCHETTE)

	Amount	% DV
Calories	110	
Fat	8 g	12%
Saturated	1 g	6%
+ Trans	0 g	
Polyunsaturated	1 g	
Omega-6	0.8 g	
Omega-3 (ALA)	0.1 g	
Omega-3 (EPA+DHA)	0 g	
Monounsaturated	5.5 g	
Cholesterol	0 mg	0%
Sodium	20 mg	1%
Potassium	436 mg	13%
Carbohydrate	10 g	4%
Dietary Fibre	2.5 g	10%
Sugars	4 g	
Protein	3 g	
Vitamin A		6%
Vitamin C		104%
Calcium		3%
Iron		7%
Vitamin D		14%
Vitamin E		17%

DIABETIC EXCHANGE

1 vegetables & fruits exchange
1 oils & fats exchange

Orange-glazed carrots

4 SERVINGS

NUTRITIONAL VALUE PER SERVING		
	Amount	% DV
Calories	85	
Fat	4 g	6%
Saturated	0.5 g	3%
+ Trans	0 g	
Polyunsaturated	0.5 g	
Omega-6	0.4 g	
Omega-3 (ALA)	0 g	
Omega-3 (EPA+DHA)	0 g	
Monounsaturated	2.5 g	
Cholesterol	0 mg	0%
Sodium	198 mg	9%
Potassium	399 mg	12%
Carbohydrate	12 g	5%
Dietary Fibre	3 g	12%
Sugars	6 g	
Protein	2 g	
Vitamin A		59%
Vitamin C		37%
Calcium		4%
Iron		4%
Vitamin D		0%
Vitamin E		12%

DIABETIC EXCHANGE

2 vegetables & fruits exchanges
1/2 oils & fats exchange

3 cups (750 ml)	carrots
	Juice and zest of one orange
2/3 cup (160 ml)	home-made chicken broth (see recipe p. 113) or fat-free salt-free commercial brand
1 tbsp.	olive oil
1/4 tsp.	salt
	Pepper to taste
1 tbsp.	chopped parsley

- Peel carrots and cut into rounds. Place in a medium-sized saucepan. Add orange juice and zest, chicken broth and oil. Season. Cook uncovered at low heat for 30 minutes.
- The liquid must be almost completely evaporated. If not, increase the heat for a few minutes. Sprinkle with parsley.

Eggplant casserole

8 SERVINGS

1	eggplant, cubed (2 cups/500 ml)
1 tbsp.	olive oil
2	sliced onions
5	tomatoes, peeled and sliced
1	cubed green pepper
1 cup (250 ml)	partially-skimmed mozzarella
1/2 tsp.	salt
	Pepper to taste
1/3 cup (80 ml)	breadcrumbs

- Cut eggplant into 1/2 inch (1 cm) thick slices, then in cubes.
- Brown in oil for 5 minutes at medium heat in a heavy non-stick frying pan.
- In an 8-cup (2-litre), lightly greased ovenproof loaf pan, alternate layers of eggplant, onion, tomato, pepper and cheese. Season each layer lightly. Mix the remaining cheese with bread-crumbs and sprinkle on top.
- Bake 1 hour at 350 °F (180 °C)

Brussels sprouts with walnuts

4 SERVINGS

NUTRITIONAL VALUE PER SERVING		
	Amount	% DV
Calories	110	
Fat	4.5 g	8%
Saturated	0.5 g	3%
+ Trans	0 g	
Polyunsaturated	2 g	
Omega-6	1.7 g	
Omega-3 (ALA)	0.5 g	
Omega-3 (EPA+DHA)	0 g	
Monounsaturated	1.5 g	
Cholesterol	0 mg	0%
Sodium	329 mg	14%
Potassium	508 mg	15%
Carbohydrate	12 g	5%
Dietary Fibre	5.5 g	22%
Sugars	3 g	
Protein	5 g	
Vitamin A		5%
Vitamin C		181%
Calcium		6%
Iron		14%
Vitamin D		0%
Vitamin E		14%

DIABETIC EXCHANGE

1 1/2 vegetables & fruits exchange
1/2 oils & fats exchange

1 lb (500 g)	Brussels sprouts
1/2 cup (125 ml)	water
1 tbsp.	lemon juice
1/2 tbsp.	olive oil
2 tbsp.	chopped walnuts
1/2 tsp.	salt
	Pepper to taste

- Trim the Brussels sprouts. Remove wilted leaves. Make an X-shaped incision at the base of each sprout so they will cook evenly. Cook over medium heat for 10 minutes in the water and lemon juice.
- In a small saucepan, heat the oil and brown the walnuts. Add well-drained Brussels sprouts. Add salt and pepper, and serve.

Crepes with asparagus filling

6 SERVINGS

NUTRITIONAL VALUE PER SERVING

	Amount	% DV
Calories	215	
Fat	8 g	12%
Saturated	2.5 g	14%
+ Trans	0.1 g	
Polyunsaturated	1 g	
Omega-6	0.7 g	
Omega-3 (ALA)	0.1 g	
Omega-3 (EPA+DHA)	0 g	
Monounsaturated	3.5 g	
Cholesterol	42 mg	14%
Sodium	392 mg	17%
Potassium	341 mg	10%
Carbohydrate	25 g	9%
Dietary Fibre	2 g	9%
Sugars	1 g	
Protein	12 g	
Vitamin A		11%
Vitamin C		14%
Calcium		22%
Iron		14%
Vitamin D		24%
Vitamin E		9%

DIABETIC EXCHANGE

1/2 milk & alternatives exchange
1/2 grain product exchange
1 vegetables & fruits exchange
2 oils & fats exchanges

CREPES:

1 recipe	Crepe batter (see recipe, p. 249)

FILLING:

12	asparagus stalks, fresh or bottled
1 1/2 tbsp.	olive oil
2 tbsp.	flour
1 cup (250 ml)	1% milk
1/2 cup (125 ml)	light swiss cheese, 15% M.F.
1/4 tsp.	salt
	Pepper to taste
1 pinch	nutmeg

- Prepare crepe batter, then prepare the crepes. Keep them warm in the oven at 150 °F (70 °C).
- If you are using fresh asparagus, cook in a very small quantity of water until the stems are tender.
- Heat the oil in a non-stick saucepan. Add flour, combine with margarine. Whisk in the milk. Cook until the mixture thickens, constantly stirring. Set aside 2 tbsp. of the cheese, adding the rest to the mixture along with salt, pepper and nutmeg. Simmer over low heat for 2 minutes, stirring.
- Arrange 2 drained asparagus stalks on each crepe and drizzle 2 tbsp. of sauce over top. Roll the crepes and place in an ovenproof dish. Pour remaining sauce over the crepes and sprinkle the rest of the grated cheese on top. Put under the grill for a few minutes until golden. Serve with a fresh green salad.

Healthy baked fries

2 SERVINGS

2	peeled potatoes
1/4 tsp.	thyme
1/4 tsp.	rosemary
1/4 tsp.	basil
1/4 tsp.	garlic powder
1/2 tsp.	paprika
1 tbsp.	olive oil
1/2 tsp.	salt

- Heat a baking sheet for 5 minutes in a preheated 400 °F (200 °C) oven.
- During this time, cut the potatoes into "fries" and put in a bowl. Add thyme, rosemary, basil, garlic powder and paprika. Combine. Sprinkle with olive oil and mix again.
- Arrange the potatoes in a single layer on the heated baking sheet. Bake at 400 °F (200 °C) for 15 minutes. Stir the fries and bake for another 15 minutes.
- Add salt and serve immediately.

NUTRITIONAL VALUE PER SERVING

	Amount	% DV
Calories	155	
Fat	7 g	11%
Saturated	1 g	5%
+ Trans	0 g	
Polyunsaturated	1 g	
Omega-6	0.8 g	
Omega-3 (ALA)	0.1 g	
Omega-3 (EPA+DHA)	0 g	
Monounsaturated	5 g	
Cholesterol	0 mg	0%
Sodium	601 mg	26%
Potassium	494 mg	15%
Carbohydrate	20 g	7%
Dietary Fibre	2 g	9%
Sugars	1 g	
Protein	3 g	
Vitamin A		2%
Vitamin C		37%
Calcium		3%
Iron		10%
Vitamin D		0%
Vitamin E		12%

DIABETIC EXCHANGE

1 1/2 grain product exchange
1 1/2 oils & fats exchange

Green beans and mushrooms with chives

6 SERVINGS

1 lb (500 g)	fresh green beans, cut in 1 inch (2.5 cm) pieces
1 tbsp.	olive oil
1	sliced onion separated into rings
2	minced garlic cloves
375 ml (1 ½ cups)	sliced white or café mushrooms
1 tbsp.	lemon juice
1 tsp.	marjoram
¼ tsp.	salt
	Pepper to taste
2 tbsp.	minced chives

- Cook beans in boiling water until tender but still crunchy. Drain and set aside.
- In a large non-stick frying pan, heat the oil. Fry onions and garlic. Add mushrooms and cook until tender. Add green beans and reheat for a few minutes, stirring.
- Add lemon juice, marjoram, salt and pepper. Sprinkle with minced chives. Serve.

NUTRITIONAL VALUE PER SERVING

	Amount	% DV
Calories	65	
Fat	2.5 g	4%
Saturated	0.5 g	2%
+ Trans	0 g	
Polyunsaturated	0.5 g	
Omega-6	0.3 g	
Omega-3 (ALA)	0.1 g	
Omega-3 (EPA+DHA)	0 g	
Monounsaturated	1.5 g	
Cholesterol	0 mg	0%
Sodium	86 mg	4%
Potassium	281 mg	9%
Carbohydrate	10 g	4%
Dietary Fibre	3.5 g	15%
Sugars	3 g	
Protein	3 g	
Vitamin A		4%
Vitamin C		30%
Calcium		4%
Iron		9%
Vitamin D		8%
Vitamin E		7%

DIABETIC EXCHANGE

1 vegetables & fruits exchange
½ oils & fats exchange

Green beans with *herbes de Provence*

4 SERVINGS

¹/₂ lb (250 g)	fresh green beans
1 tbsp.	olive oil
¹/₂ cup (125 ml)	spanish onion, cut and separated into rings
1	finely minced garlic clove
¹/₄ cup (60 ml)	red pepper cut into little cubes
¹/₄ tsp.	*herbes de Provence* (see recipe, p. 259)
¹/₄ cup (60 ml)	water
¹/₄ tsp.	salt
	Pepper to taste
1 tbsp.	chopped chives

- Prepare beans by cutting them French-style, that is, into thin strips. Heat the oil in a large non-stick frying pan. Fry onion and garlic for 5 minutes, until soft. Add remaining ingredients except for chives.
- Cover and simmer for 5 minutes. Add chives.

NUTRITIONAL VALUE PER SERVING

	Amount	% DV
Calories	50	
Fat	2.5 g	4%
Saturated	0.5 g	2%
+ Trans	0 g	
Polyunsaturated	0.5 g	
Omega-6	0.3 g	
Omega-3 (ALA)	0.1 g	
Omega-3 (EPA+DHA)	0 g	
Monounsaturated	1.5 g	
Cholesterol	0 mg	0%
Sodium	83 mg	4%
Potassium	121 mg	4%
Carbohydrate	5 g	2%
Dietary Fibre	1.5 g	7%
Sugars	2 g	
Protein	1 g	
Vitamin A		3%
Vitamin C		34%
Calcium		2%
Iron		4%
Vitamin D		0%
Vitamin E		7%

DIABETIC EXCHANGE

1 vegetables & fruits exchange
1 oils & fats exchange

Winter vegetables julienne

4 SERVINGS

1 tsp.	olive oil
2	carrots, peeled and cut into fine strips
1	parsnip, peeled and cut into fine strips
2	very finely minced garlic cloves
1	minced dried shallot
1 tsp.	poppy seeds
1	zucchini cut into fine strips
3	celery stalks cut into fine strips
1/4 cup (60 ml)	home-made chicken broth (see recipe, p. 113) or fat-free salt-free commercial broth
1/4 tsp.	salt
	Pepper to taste

- Heat the oil in a large non-stick frying pan. Add carrots, parsnips, garlic and shallot. Cook stirring for 3 minutes. Add poppy seeds, zucchini and celery. Cook for 3 more minutes, stirring.
- Add chicken broth and season. Cover and cook for another 5 minutes. The vegetables should still be crunchy. Serve immediately.

NUTRITIONAL VALUE PER SERVING

	Amount	% DV
Calories	85	
Fat	4 g	7%
Saturated	0.5 g	3%
+ Trans	0 g	
Polyunsaturated	0.5 g	
Omega-6	0.6 g	
Omega-3 (ALA)	0.1 g	
Omega-3 (EPA+DHA)	0 g	
Monounsaturated	2.5 g	
Cholesterol	0 mg	0%
Sodium	190 mg	8%
Potassium	447 mg	13%
Carbohydrate	11 g	4%
Dietary Fibre	3 g	12%
Sugars	4 g	
Protein	2 g	
Vitamin A		26%
Vitamin C		27%
Calcium		6%
Iron		5%
Vitamin D		0%
Vitamin E		13%

DIABETIC EXCHANGE

2 vegetables & fruits exchanges
1/2 oils & fats exchange

Vegetable stir-fry

6 SERVINGS

NUTRITIONAL VALUE PER SERVING

	Amount	% DV
Calories	95	
Fat	5 g	9%
Saturated	0.5 g	4%
+ Trans	0 g	
Polyunsaturated	1 g	
Omega-6	0.7 g	
Omega-3 (ALA)	0.1 g	
Omega-3 (EPA+DHA)	0 g	
Monounsaturated	3.5 g	
Cholesterol	1 mg	1%
Sodium	198 mg	9%
Potassium	355 mg	11%
Carbohydrate	12 g	4%
Dietary Fibre	2.5 g	10%
Sugars	4 g	
Protein	2 g	
Vitamin A		15%
Vitamin C		102%
Calcium		4%
Iron		5%
Vitamin D		0%
Vitamin E		11%

DIABETIC EXCHANGE

2 vegetables & fruits exchanges
1 oils & fats exchange

2 tbsp.	olive oil
1	spanish onion cut in large cubes
2	minced garlic cloves
1 tbsp.	fresh ginger, finely chopped
1 cup (250 ml)	sliced carrots
1 cup (250 ml)	cauliflower flowerets
1 cup (250 ml)	broccoli flowerets
1 cup (250 ml)	celery, sliced diagonally
1/2	yellow pepper cut in fine strips
1/2	green pepper cut in fine strips
2/3 cup (160 ml)	home-made chicken broth (see recipe, p. 113) or fat-free salt-free commercial broth
2 tbsp.	cold water
2 tsp.	cornstarch
1 tbsp.	light soya sauce
1/2 tsp.	sesame oil
1 tbsp.	hoisin sauce

- Heat the oil in a wok or a large non-stick frying pan. Sauté onion, garlic and ginger for 2 minutes. Add carrots, cauliflower, broccoli, celery and two colours of peppers. Stir-fry for 3 minutes.
- Add chicken broth, cover pan and steam for 5 minutes. In a small bowl, mix water, cornstarch, soya sauce, sesame oil and hoisin sauce. Clear a space in the middle of the wok and add cornstarch mixture to sauce. Stir until it thickens. Mix well so that all the vegetables are coated in sauce. Serve.

Vegetables en papillote

4 SERVINGS

(COOKED ON THE BARBECUE)

4	medium-sized potatoes, cubed
4	medium-sized carrots, sliced
2	medium-sized onions cut in rings
2	zucchini cut in rounds
1	red pepper cut in large squares
1/2 tsp.	salt
1/4 tsp.	pepper
1 tsp.	chopped fresh basil
1 tsp.	chopped fresh savory
1 tbsp.	olive oil

- Prepare all the vegetables and spread over 2 sheets of aluminium foil sprayed with no-stick vegetable spray. Add to each half, in equal parts: salt, pepper, basil, savory and oil.
- Fold the edges of the foil, carefully sealing "papillotes" (foil packets) so that no steam can escape. Place on the barbecue grill. Cook for 20 minutes turning papillotes over every 5 minutes.

NUTRITIONAL VALUE PER SERVING

	Amount	% DV
Calories	170	
Fat	4 g	6%
Saturated	0.5 g	3%
+ Trans	0 g	
Polyunsaturated	1 g	
Omega-6	0.5 g	
Omega-3 (ALA)	0.1 g	
Omega-3 (EPA+DHA)	0 g	
Monounsaturated	2.5 g	
Cholesterol	0 mg	0%
Sodium	361 mg	16%
Potassium	787 mg	23%
Carbohydrate	32 g	11%
Dietary Fibre	4.5 g	18%
Sugars	7 g	
Protein	4 g	
Vitamin A		49%
Vitamin C		48%
Calcium		5%
Iron		10%
Vitamin D		0%
Vitamin E		11%

DIABETIC EXCHANGE

2 vegetables & fruits exchanges
1 1/2 grain product exchange
1/2 oils & fats exchange

Small pizzas with vegetables

MAKES 4 PIZZAS

(COOKED ON THE BARBECUE)

	Margarine
8 slices	whole-wheat bread
1/2 cup (125 ml)	tomato sauce (see recipe, p. 212)
1/2 tsp.	garlic powder
1/2 tsp.	oregano
1/4	finely sliced green pepper
1/4	finely sliced red pepper
4	large sliced mushrooms
1/2	small sliced zucchini
1/4 cup (60 ml)	red onion cut into rings
1/2 cup (125 ml)	partially-skimmed grated mozzarella

- Spread a thin layer of margarine on one side of each slice of bread. Next, on the side without margarine, spread tomato sauce, and season with garlic powder and oregano. Arrange vegetables and mozzarella on these 4 slices. Cover with the other slices, and spread margarine on the outside.
- Heat barbecue to medium-high and place pizzas on a rack above the barbecue grill. Cook until golden. Turn the pizzas over and cook on the other side.
- The pizzas can also be made in a large non-stick frying pan on the stove-top.
- These little improvised pizzas are appreciated by grownups and kids alike.

NUTRITIONAL VALUE PER SERVING

	Amount	% DV
Calories	210	
Fat	5 g	8%
v	2 g	11%
+ Trans	0 g	
Polyunsaturated	1 g	
Omega-6	0.7 g	
Omega-3 (ALA)	0.1 g	
Omega-3 (EPA+DHA)	0 g	
Monounsaturated	1.5 g	
Cholesterol	9 mg	3%
Sodium	378 mg	16%
Potassium	462 mg	14%
Carbohydrate	33 g	11%
Dietary Fibre	5.5 g	22%
Sugars	15 g	
Protein	11 g	
Vitamin A		5%
Vitamin C		79%
Calcium		14%
Iron		19%
Vitamin D		9%
Vitamin E		12%

DIABETIC EXCHANGE

1 vegetables & fruits exchange
2 grain product exchanges
1 1/3 oils & fats exchange

Asparagus roll-ups

MAKES 12 SMALL SANDWICHES

12 slices	whole-wheat bread
1/2 cup (125 ml)	yogourt cheese (see recipe, p. 108)
3/4 lb (350 g)	bottled asparagus spears, drained

- Remove bread crusts. Spread each slice with yogourt cheese.
- Place an asparagus spear on each slice. Roll up tightly and arrange on a serving platter.
- Cover with a damp cloth. Refrigerate. Do not keep the roll-ups longer than 5 hours, for they will get soggy.

NUTRITIONAL VALUE PER SERVING

	Amount	% DV
Calories	85	
Fat	1.5 g	3%
Saturated	0.5 g	2%
+ Trans	0 g	
Polyunsaturated	0.5 g	
Omega-6	0.4 g	
Omega-3 (ALA)	0.1 g	
Omega-3 (EPA+DHA)	0 g	
Monounsaturated	0.5 g	
Cholesterol	1 mg	1%
Sodium	229 mg	10%
Potassium	141 mg	5%
Carbohydrate	15 g	5%
Dietary Fibre	2.5 g	10%
Sugars	7 g	
Protein	4 g	
Vitamin A		2%
Vitamin C		8%
Calcium		4%
Iron		11%
Vitamin D		1%
Vitamin E		2%

DIABETIC EXCHANGE

1 grain product exchange

Summer vegetable sandwiches (bruschettas)

2 SERVINGS

4 slices	whole wheat baguette
1 cup (250 ml)	fresh tomatoes, seeded and diced
2	minced garlic cloves
2	sliced green onions
1/4 cup (60 ml)	diced yellow peppers
1/3 cup (80 ml)	light Emmenthal 15% M.F., grated
2 tbsp.	fresh basil, chopped fine
1/2 tsp.	salt
	Pepper to taste

- Heat oven to 400 °F (200 °C).
- Cut 4 diagonal slices of baguette, 3/4 inch (2 cm) thick.
- Mix other ingredients. Spread mixture on the slices of bread and bake in oven for 10 to 12 minutes, or until cheese is melted. Serve hot.

NUTRITIONAL VALUE PER SERVING

	Amount	% DV
Calories	175	
Fat	5.5 g	9%
Saturated	2.5 g	14%
+ Trans	0 g	
Polyunsaturated	1 g	
Omega-6	0.6 g	
Omega-3 (ALA)	0.1 g	
Omega-3 (EPA+DHA)	0 g	
Monounsaturated	1.5 g	
Cholesterol	13 mg	5%
Sodium	865 mg	37%
Potassium	422 mg	13%
Carbohydrate	22 g	8%
Dietary Fibre	3.5 g	14%
Sugars	6 g	
Protein	10 g	
Vitamin A		9%
Vitamin C		88%
Calcium		17%
Iron		14%
Vitamin D		0%
Vitamin E		5%

DIABETIC EXCHANGE

1 vegetables & fruits exchange
2 grain product exchanges
1/2 meat & alternatives exchange

147

Meat and poultry

Grilled lamp chops

4 SERVINGS

(BARBECUE OR TRADITIONAL METHOD)

8	**lamp chops 1 inch (2.5 cm) thick, with as much fat removed as possible**

MARINADE:

¹/₄ cup (60 ml)	raspberry vinegar
2	chopped dried shallots
2	minced garlic cloves
¹/₄ cup (60 ml)	chopped celery
¹/₄ tsp.	rosemary
¹/₄ tsp.	basil
2 tbsp.	olive oil
¹/₂ tsp.	salt
	Pepper to taste

- Place lamb chops side by side in a shallow dish.
- In a small bowl, combine vinegar, shallot, garlic, celery, rosemary, basil, oil, salt and pepper. Pour over lamb chops. Marinate in the refrigerator for at least 2 hours, turning the chops 2 or 3 times in the marinade.
- Remove lamb chops from refrigerator ¹/₂ hour before cooking.
- Heat the barbecue to medium-high, or turn on the oven broiler. Place lamb chops on a grill and cook at a distance of 4 to 6 inches (10 to 15 cm) from the heat source, 3 ¹/₂ to 4 minutes each side. The meat, as seen through a small cut in the centre of one of the chops, should still be slightly pink.
- Serve with mint sauce (see recipe, p. 209).

NUTRITIONAL VALUE PER SERVING

	Amount	% DV
Calories	230	
Fat	13 g	21%
Saturated	4.5 g	22%
+ Trans	0 g	
Polyunsaturated	1 g	
Omega-6	0.9 g	
Omega-3 (ALA)	0.2 g	
Omega-3 (EPA+DHA)	0 g	
Monounsaturated	6 g	
Cholesterol	83 mg	28%
Sodium	150 mg	7%
Potassium	346 mg	10%
Carbohydrate	1 g	1%
Dietary Fibre	0 g	1%
Sugars	0 g	
Protein	25 g	
Vitamin A		1%
Vitamin C		1%
Calcium		2%
Iron		16%
Vitamin D		10%
Vitamin E		5%

DIABETIC EXCHANGE

3 meat & alternatives exchanges
¹/₂ oils & fats exchange

Delicious leg of lamb

8 SERVINGS

1	fresh leg of lamb, about 3 lbs (1.5 kg)
2	garlic cloves
1/2 tsp.	salt
	Pepper to taste
1 1/4 cup (310 ml)	home-made beef broth (see recipe p. 112) or no-fat no-salt commercial broth
1 cup (250 ml)	fresh sliced mushrooms
3	chopped green onions
1	chopped stalk of celery
1 tsp.	fresh finely chopped ginger
1 tbsp.	low-sodium soya sauce
1 tsp.	dried mint
1/2 tsp.	basil
2 tbsp.	cornstarch
1/4 cup (60 ml)	water

- Completely remove fat from leg of lamb. Cut garlic cloves in two and insert them in the meat. Place the leg of lamb in a shallow roasting pan and cook uncovered for 1 1/2 hours at 325 °F (160 °C). Halfway through cooking, add salt and pepper.
- Pour out fat, if any, from the roasting pan.
- Mix beef broth, mushrooms, green onions, celery, ginger, soya sauce, mint and basil. Pour over the lamb. Cook for another 45 minutes basting 2 or 3 times.
- When the meat is cooked, remove it from the roasting pan and keep warm.
- Mix the cornstarch with water. Add broth and finish cooking on the stove-top, stirring until the mixture thickens. Carve, and serve lamb slices with sauce poured over top.

NUTRITIONAL VALUE PER SERVING

	Amount	% DV
Calories	180	
Fat	6 g	9%
Saturated	2 g	11%
+ Trans	0 g	
Polyunsaturated	0.5 g	
Omega-6	0.4 g	
Omega-3 (ALA)	0.1 g	
Omega-3 (EPA+DHA)	0 g	
Monounsaturated	2.5 g	
Cholesterol	80 mg	27%
Sodium	319 mg	14%
Potassium	468 mg	14%
Carbohydrate	4 g	2%
Dietary Fibre	0.5 g	2%
Sugars	0 g	
Protein	27 g	
Vitamin A		1%
Vitamin C		6%
Calcium		2%
Iron		19%
Vitamin D		9%
Vitamin E		3%

DIABETIC EXCHANGE

3 meat & alternatives exchanges

Pan-fried sliced lamb

4 SERVINGS

NUTRITIONAL VALUE PER SERVING

	Amount	% DV
Calories	225	
Fat	9 g	15%
Saturated	2.5 g	13%
+ Trans	0 g	
Polyunsaturated	1 g	
Omega-6	0.8 g	
Omega-3 (ALA)	0.1 g	
Omega-3 (EPA+DHA)	0 g	
Monounsaturated	5 g	
Cholesterol	80 mg	27%
Sodium	404 mg	17%
Potassium	627 mg	18%
Carbohydrate	7 g	3%
Dietary Fibre	1.5 g	6%
Sugars	3 g	
Protein	28 g	
Vitamin A		2%
Vitamin C		9%
Calcium		4%
Iron		24%
Vitamin D		13%
Vitamin E		13%

DIABETIC EXCHANGE

1/2 vegetables & fruits exchange
4 meat & alternatives exchanges
1/2 oils & fats exchange

4	slices of leg of lamb, 7 oz (200 g) each
1 tbsp.	olive oil
1	finely sliced onion
1	crushed garlic clove
1 cup (250 ml)	home-made beef broth (see recipe, p. 112) or fat-free salt-free commercial broth
2 tbsp.	tomato paste
1 tbsp.	balsamic vinegar
1 tsp.	oregano
1 tbsp.	finely chopped fresh mint, or 1 tsp. dried mint
1 cup (250 ml)	fresh mushrooms cut in quarters
1/2 tsp.	salt
	Pepper to taste

- Remove all fat from sliced lamb. In a large non-stick frying pan, heat oil. Fry lamb slices on both sides until golden. Remove from pan, set aside.
- In the same frying pan, brown onion and garlic. Add beef broth, tomato paste, balsamic vinegar, oregano and mint. Add lamb slices, cover and simmer over low heat for 1/2 hour.
- Add mushrooms and cook over very low heat for another 1/2 hour. Season, serve.

Beef bourguignon

6 SERVINGS

NUTRITIONAL VALUE PER SERVING

	Amount	% DV
Calories	360	
Fat	14 g	23%
Saturated	4.5 g	24%
+ Trans	0 g	
Polyunsaturated	1 g	
Omega-6	0.8 g	
Omega-3 (ALA)	0.1 g	
Omega-3 (EPA+DHA)	0 g	
Monounsaturated	6 g	
Cholesterol	82 mg	28%
Sodium	531 mg	23%
Potassium	1051 mg	31%
Carbohydrate	11 g	4%
Dietary Fibre	1 g	5%
Sugars	3 g	
Protein	39 g	
Vitamin A		14%
Vitamin C		12%
Calcium		4%
Iron		31%
Vitamin D		27%
Vitamin E		5%

DIABETIC EXCHANGE

1 vegetables & fruits exchange
5 meat & alternatives exchanges
1 oils & fats exchange

1 tbsp.	olive oil
2 lb (1 kg)	very lean beef in 1 inch (2.5 cm) cubes
1/4 cup (60 ml)	flour
3	chopped green onions
2	minced garlic cloves
1 cup (250 ml)	home-made chicken broth (see recipe, p. 113) or fat-free salt-free commercial broth
1 cup (250 ml)	dry red wine
1 tsp.	salt
1/4 tsp.	pepper
1 cup (250 ml)	carrots cut in rounds
1 cup (250 ml)	small onions
1 cup (250 ml)	small mushrooms

- Preheat oven to 350 °F (180 °C). Heat oil in a large non-stick frying pan.
- Coat beef cubes with flour, and brown in the frying pan. Transfer to an oven-proof casserole. In the frying pan, cook green onions and garlic until golden. Add to the meat in the casserole, then add chicken broth and red wine. Cover casserole, place in oven and bake for 2 1/2 hours. One hour before the end of cooking, season. Add carrots and little onions. Half an hour before the end of cooking, add mushrooms.

Beef daube provençale

8 SERVINGS

NUTRITIONAL VALUE PER SERVING

	Amount	% DV
Calories	395	
Fat	18 g	28%
Saturated	5.5 g	28%
+ Trans	0 g	
Polyunsaturated	1 g	
Omega-6	1.1 g	
Omega-3 (ALA)	0.1 g	
Omega-3 (EPA+DHA)	0 g	
Monounsaturated	8 g	
Cholesterol	92 mg	31%
Sodium	517 mg	22%
Potassium	1255 mg	36%
Carbohydrate	9 g	3%
Dietary Fibre	2 g	9%
Sugars	3 g	
Protein	44 g	
Vitamin A		15%
Vitamin C		18%
Calcium		5%
Iron		35%
Vitamin D		27%
Vitamin E		12%

DIABETIC EXCHANGE

1 vegetables & fruits exchange
6 meat & alternatives exchanges
1 oils & fats exchange

2 tbsp.	olive oil
3 lb (1.5 kg)	lean beef cut into 1 ½ inch (4 cm) cubes
1	onion sliced into rings
2	chopped garlic cloves
2	carrots cut in rounds
2 cups (500 ml)	home-made beef broth (see recipe, p. 112) or fat-free salt-free commercial broth
1 cup (250 ml)	dry red wine
3 tbsp.	tomato paste
1	bouquet garni made of 2 sprigs of parsley, 1 sprig of thyme, 1 bay leaf (tied together with a piece of string)
5	peppercorns
1	whole onion studded with 5 cloves
	Zest of 1 orange
1 tsp.	salt
1 cup (250 ml)	halved mushrooms
3	tomatoes, blanched, peeled and cubed
½ cup (125 ml)	small black olives, rinsed

- Preheat oven to 325 °F (160 °C). Heat the oil in a large non-stick frying pan. Brown meat on all sides. Set aside.
- In the same frying pan, brown onion, garlic and carrots for 5 minutes at medium heat then transfer with the meat to a large casserole. Add broth, wine and tomato paste. Tie together thyme, bay leaf and parsley. Put peppercorns in a little square of cheesecloth and tie it up. Place the bouquet garni among the meat cubes, along with the clove-studded onion and orange zest. Add salt.
- Cover casserole and bake for 3 hours. Half an hour before the end of cooking, add mushrooms, tomatoes and black olives. At the end of cooking, remove the bouquet garni, pepper, whole onion and orange zest.

Beef brochettes

4 SERVINGS

(BARBECUE OR TRADITIONAL METHOD)

NUTRITIONAL VALUE PER SERVING

	Amount	% DV
Calories	285	
Fat	10 g	16%
Saturated	3 g	15%
+ Trans	0 g	
Polyunsaturated	0.5 g	
Omega-6	0.6 g	
Omega-3 (ALA)	0 g	
Omega-3 (EPA+DHA)	0 g	
Monounsaturated	5 g	
Cholesterol	91 mg	31%
Sodium	158 mg	7%
Potassium	691 mg	20%
Carbohydrate	6 g	3%
Dietary Fibre	1 g	5%
Sugars	3 g	
Protein	40 g	
Vitamin A		1%
Vitamin C		33%
Calcium		4%
Iron		20%
Vitamin D		17%
Vitamin E		11%

DIABETIC EXCHANGE

3 meat & alternatives exchanges
1/2 vegetables & fruits exchange
1/2 oils & fats exchange

MARINADE:

1/2 cup (125 ml)	red wine
1/4 cup (60 ml)	olive oil
1/2 tsp.	Worcestershire sauce
1	chopped garlic clove
1 tbsp.	tomato ketchup
1/2 tsp.	salt
1 tbsp.	balsamic vinegar
1/2 tsp.	rosemary
1/2 tsp.	marjoram
1 lb (500 g)	sirloin steak cut in 20 cubes, fat removed
1/2	green pepper cut in 8 pieces
4	mushrooms
1	onion cut in quarters

- Mix all marinade ingredients. Place beef pieces in marinade. Marinate 2 hours at room temperature.
- Blanch vegetables 1 minute. Drain beef and prepare brochettes, alternating vegetables with 5 cubes of beef per brochette.
- Depending on the season, cook on the barbecue or under the broiler, 10 cm (4 inches) from the heat source, for 6 to 8 minutes or until meat is done to your liking. Halfway through cooking, turn the brochettes and baste with marinade. Serve with Vegetable rice or Rice ring with fine herbs (see recipes p. 129 and 130).
- These brochettes are delicious when served with Mushroom sauce (see recipe, p. 208). If you are serving this sauce with the brochettes, make it with 1 cup (250 ml) of beef broth instead of 3/4 cup (180 ml).

Quick & tasty meatloaf

6 SERVINGS

1 ½ lb (750 g)	extra-lean ground beef
3 cups (750 ml)	crustless whole wheat bread, cubed
⅓ cup (80 ml)	stuffed olives, rinsed with water and chopped
¾ tsp.	salt
¼ tsp.	pepper
1	finely chopped onion
1	egg, lightly beaten
½ cup (125 ml)	hot water
1 cup (250 ml)	chopped celery
¼ tsp.	paprika
2 tbsp.	olive oil
1 pinch	savory

- Preheat oven to 350 °F (180 °C).
- Crumble meat with a fork and add all other ingredients, in the order given above. Combine well. Place in a bread pan sprayed with non-stick vegetable spray. Bake for 1 hour.

Note This meatloaf is very good served hot with Tomato sauce (see recipe, p. 212) or Mushroom sauce (see recipe, p. 208). If there is any left over, serve cold as a paté with crackers.

NUTRITIONAL VALUE PER SERVING

	Amount	% DV
Calories	340	
Fat	16 g	25%
Saturated	5 g	27%
+ Trans	0.3 g	
Polyunsaturated	1.5 g	
Omega-6	1.1 g	
Omega-3 (ALA)	0.2 g	
Omega-3 (EPA+DHA)	0.1 g	
Monounsaturated	9 g	
Cholesterol	100 mg	34%
Sodium	517 mg	22%
Potassium	539 mg	16%
Carbohydrate	17 g	6%
Dietary Fibre	3 g	12%
Sugars	8 g	
Protein	31 g	
Vitamin A		2%
Vitamin C		4%
Calcium		5%
Iron		28%
Vitamin D		8%
Vitamin E		14%

DIABETIC EXCHANGE

½ vegetables & fruits exchange
½ grain product exchange
4 meat & alternatives exchange
1 oils & fats exchange

Mini-meatloaf

6 SERVINGS

NUTRITIONAL VALUE PER SERVING		
	Amount	% DV
Calories	215	
Fat	8 g	13%
Saturated	3.5 g	18%
+ Trans	0.2 g	
Polyunsaturated	0.5 g	
Omega-6	0.3 g	
Omega-3 (ALA)	0.1 g	
Omega-3 (EPA+DHA)	0 g	
Monounsaturated	3.5 g	
Cholesterol	70 mg	24%
Sodium	330 mg	14%
Potassium	447 mg	13%
Carbohydrate	12 g	4%
Dietary Fibre	1.5 g	6%
Sugars	3 g	
Protein	24 g	
Vitamin A		4%
Vitamin C		25%
Calcium		6%
Iron		15%
Vitamin D		18%
Vitamin E		5%

DIABETIC EXCHANGE

1/2 grain product exchange
3 meat & alternatives exchanges

2	Shredded Wheat biscuits
5 oz (150 ml)	1% milk
3/4 lb (375 g)	extra-lean ground beef
1/2 lb (250 g)	ground veal
1	lightly beaten egg
1/4 cup (60 ml)	chopped onion
1/4 cup (60 ml)	celery with leaves, finely chopped
2 tbsp.	red pepper, diced fine
1 tbsp.	ketchup
1/2 tsp.	salt
1/2 tsp.	oregano
	Pepper to taste
2 tbsp.	chopped parsley
	Mushroom sauce (see recipe, p. 208)

- Crumble Shredded Wheat biscuits in a bowl. Add milk and let sit for 5 minutes. Add meat, egg, vegetables, ketchup and seasonings. Mix well.
- Form 6 big meatballs. Distribute in a muffin pan sprayed with non-stick vegetable spray.
- Bake at 350 °F (180 °C) for 30 minutes or until meat is cooked inside. Serve with the mushroom sauce.

Pot-au-feu (beef stew)

6 SERVINGS

(COOKED IN A PRESSURE-COOKER)

NUTRITIONAL VALUE PER SERVING		
	Amount	% DV
Calories	305	
Fat	12 g	18%
Saturated	3.5 g	18%
+ Trans	0 g	
Polyunsaturated	1 g	
Omega-6	0.7 g	
Omega-3 (ALA)	0.1 g	
Omega-3 (EPA+DHA)	0 g	
Monounsaturated	5 g	
Cholesterol	62 mg	21%
Sodium	553 mg	24%
Potassium	1172 mg	34%
Carbohydrate	20 g	7%
Dietary Fibre	4.5 g	19%
Sugars	7 g	
Protein	32 g	
Vitamin A		27%
Vitamin C		49%
Calcium		9%
Iron		29%
Vitamin D		15%
Vitamin E		16%

1 tbsp.	olive oil
1 1/2 lb (750 g)	beef, cut in cubes with fat removed
2	chopped onions
1	bay leaf
1 tsp.	oregano
2 cups (500 ml)	home-made beef broth (see recipe, p. 112) or fat-free salt-free commercial broth
2 tbsp.	tomato paste
1 tsp.	salt
1/4 tsp.	pepper
3	carrots, thickly sliced
2	parsnips, thickly sliced
1	turnip cut in large cubes
1/2	cabbage with a string tied around it to prevent it from falling apart
	Green and yellow beans mixed, tied in bunches for individual servings.

- Heat oil in a large non-stick frying pan. Brown beef cubes on all sides. Remove meat from pan and transfer to the pressure-cooker.
- In the same frying pan, brown onion for 3 minutes, stirring. Add meat with bay leaf and oregano. Mix beef broth and tomato paste, pour over meat. Put the lid on the pressure-cooker and cook for 20 minutes. Cool the pressure-cooker under cold water.
- When the pressure has subsided, open pressure-cooker. Sprinkle salt and pepper on the meat. Add vegetables. Close the lid again and cook for another 10 minutes.
- Remove from heat and let the pressure subside on its own.

DIABETIC EXCHANGE

3 vegetables exchanges
4 meat & alternatives exchanges
1/2 oils & fats exchange

Roast beef on the embers

6 SERVINGS

(COOKED ON BARBECUE)

NUTRITIONAL VALUE PER SERVING

	Amount	% DV
Calories	380	
Fat	17 g	26%
Saturated	6.5 g	33%
+ Trans	0 g	
Polyunsaturated	1.5 g	
Omega-6	1.1 g	
Omega-3 (ALA)	0.1 g	
Omega-3 (EPA+DHA)	0 g	
Monounsaturated	9 g	
Cholesterol	123 mg	41%
Sodium	339 mg	15%
Potassium	1102 mg	32%
Carbohydrate	2 g	1%
Dietary Fibre	0 g	1%
Sugars	1 g	
Protein	54 g	
Vitamin A		1%
Vitamin C		1%
Calcium		3%
Iron		33%
Vitamin D		30%
Vitamin E		6%

DIABETIC EXCHANGE

6 meat & alternatives exchanges
1 1/2 oils & fats exchange

MARINADE:

1 cup (250 ml)	red wine
2 tbsp.	low-sodium soya sauce
3 tbsp.	olive oil
1	crumbled bay leaf
1	finely chopped shallot
2	minced garlic cloves
1 tbsp.	chopped fresh ginger
1/2 tsp.	crushed coriander seed
10	crushed peppercorns
1/2 tsp.	salt
2 tbsp.	finely chopped fresh rosemary

3 lb (1.5 kg)	beef roast

- The day before, mix together the marinade ingredients. If the roast is wrapped in a layer of fat, remove it and discard. Firmly tie with butcher's string.
- Place roast in a thick plastic bag. Pour marinade over meat. Expel air from the bag and carefully seal. Place in a big bowl and refrigerate overnight.
- Just before cooking, remove roast from the marinade. Drain well and slide onto the roasting spit.
- Place a drip pan filled with water on the coals under the roast. Keep an eye on the water level throughout cooking. It will prevent the formation of flames.
- Close the barbecue lid and cook at medium-high: 13 minutes per pound (500 g) for a rare roast, 18 minutes for medium and 20 minutes for well-done.
- The roast will be delicious served with Vegetables en papillote (see recipe, p. 142), placed on the coals 20 minutes before the end of cooking time. Serve immediately.

Barbecue pork chops

6 SERVINGS

6	pork chops, 3/4 inch (2 cm) thick and weighing 5 oz (150 g) each
2 tbsp.	flour
1 tbsp.	olive oil
1 tbsp.	Dijon mustard
1	small chopped onion
1 tbsp.	Worcestershire sauce
1/2 cup (125 ml)	tomato juice
1/4 cup (60 ml)	water
2 tbsp.	ketchup
2 tbsp.	wine vinegar
1/4 tsp.	ground cloves
1/2 tsp.	salt
	Pepper to taste

- Remove all visible fat from the pork chops. Lightly coat with flour. Heat oil in a large non-stick frying pan. Brown pork chops on either side.
- Mix all other ingredients and pour over meat. Reduce heat and simmer on low heat until chops are tender, about 1 hour. Add a little water if necessary.

NUTRITIONAL VALUE PER SERVING

	Amount	% DV
Calories	225	
Fat	6 g	10%
Saturated	1.5 g	8%
+ Trans	0 g	
Polyunsaturated	1 g	
Omega-6	0.4 g	
Omega-3 (ALA)	0.1 g	
Omega-3 (EPA+DHA)	0 g	
Monounsaturated	3 g	
Cholesterol	83 mg	28%
Sodium	651 mg	28%
Potassium	842 mg	25%
Carbohydrate	7 g	3%
Dietary Fibre	0.5 g	3%
Sugars	4 g	
Protein	35 g	
Vitamin A		1%
Vitamin C		7%
Calcium		3%
Iron		10%
Vitamin D		3%
Vitamin E		8%

DIABETIC EXCHANGE

4 meat & alternatives exchanges
1/2 oils & fats exchange

Hawaiian pork chops

4 SERVINGS

NUTRITIONAL VALUE PER SERVING

	Amount	% DV
Calories	350	
Fat	4 g	6%
Saturated	1 g	6%
+ Trans	0 g	
Polyunsaturated	0.5 g	
Omega-6	0.1 g	
Omega-3 (ALA)	0 g	
Omega-3 (EPA+DHA)	0 g	
Monounsaturated	1.5 g	
Cholesterol	83 mg	28%
Sodium	491 mg	21%
Potassium	991 mg	29%
Carbohydrate	39 g	13%
Dietary Fibre	1.5 g	7%
Sugars	9 g	
Protein	37 g	
Vitamin A		1%
Vitamin C		67%
Calcium		6%
Iron		12%
Vitamin D		3%
Vitamin E		5%

DIABETIC EXCHANGE

3 meat & alternatives exchanges
2 grain product exchanges
1/2 vegetables & fruits exchange

4	pork chops, 3/4 inch (2 cm) thick, fat removed
1/4 cup (60 ml)	water
1/4 tsp.	salt
1 cup (250 ml)	home-made chicken broth (see recipe p. 113) or fat-free salt-free commercial broth
2 tbsp.	cornstarch
1/2 cup (125 ml)	unsweetened pineapple juice
1/2 tsp.	Worcestershire sauce
1 tsp.	low-sodium soya sauce
1 tbsp.	vinegar
1/4 tsp.	Dijon mustard
1 cup (250 ml)	unsweetened pineapple cubes
1/2	green pepper cut in cubes
2	sliced celery stalks
2 cups (500 ml)	cooked rice, long-grain white or brown
	Pepper to taste

- Remove all visible fat from chops. Brown in a large non-stick frying pan without fat. Add 1/4 cup (60 ml) water and salt. Cover and simmer on low for about 40 minutes.
- Remove chops and keep warm. Mix chicken broth and cornstarch. Transfer to frying pan. Add pineapple juice, Worcestershire sauce, soya sauce, vinegar and mustard. Simmer until mixture thickens.
- Return chops to sauce, add pineapple cubes, green pepper and celery. Simmer for another 5 minutes. Add pepper to taste. Serve on a bed of rice.

Double-boiler turkey dressing

12 SERVINGS

NUTRITIONAL VALUE PER SERVING		
	Amount	**% DV**
Calories	120	
Fat	8 g	12%
Saturated	3 g	14%
+ Trans	0 g	
Polyunsaturated	1 g	
Omega-6	0.7 g	
Omega-3 (ALA)	0 g	
Omega-3 (EPA+DHA)	0 g	
Monounsaturated	3.5 g	
Cholesterol	24 mg	8%
Sodium	197 mg	9%
Potassium	153 mg	5%
Carbohydrate	6 g	2%
Dietary Fibre	1 g	4%
Sugars	2 g	
Protein	7 g	
Vitamin A		1%
Vitamin C		2%
Calcium		2%
Iron		6%
Vitamin D		4%
Vitamin E		2%

DIABETIC EXCHANGE
1 1/2 meat & alternatives exchange
1/2 oils & fats exchange

1 lb (500 g)	lean chopped pork
2 cups (500 ml)	crustless whole-wheat bread cut into small cubes
10	stuffed olives, rinsed in cold water and chopped
1/8 tsp.	pepper
1	small finely chopped onion
80 ml (1/3 cup)	hot water
180 ml (3/4 cup)	chopped celery
1/2 tsp.	salt
1/4 tsp.	paprika
1 pinch	savory

- Cook pork in a non-stick frying pan, and drain excess fat.
- When the meat is cooked, place in the top part of a double boiler and add remaining stuffing ingredients.
- Cook at low heat for 1 1/2 to 2 hours. Stuffing can be prepared ahead of time and reheated.

Pork tenderloin with cranberries

6 SERVINGS

NUTRITIONAL VALUE PER SERVING		
	Amount	% DV
Calories	280	
Fat	7 g	11%
Saturated	2 g	10%
+ Trans	0 g	
Polyunsaturated	1 g	
Omega-6	0.7 g	
Omega-3 (ALA)	0.1 g	
Omega-3 (EPA+DHA)	0 g	
Monounsaturated	3.5 g	
Cholesterol	99 mg	33%
Sodium	343 mg	15%
Potassium	723 mg	21%
Carbohydrate	13 g	5%
Dietary Fibre	2 g	8%
Sugars	8 g	
Protein	42 g	
Vitamin A		1%
Vitamin C		8%
Calcium		3%
Iron		20%
Vitamin D		4%
Vitamin E		5%

DIABETIC EXCHANGE

1/2 vegetables & fruits exchange
5 meat & alternatives exchanges

1 tbsp.	olive oil
2 tbsp.	onion, finely chopped
2 tbsp.	celery, finely chopped
1	cooking apple, peeled and cored, cut in cubes
3 tbsp.	currants
1/2 cup (125 ml)	raw chopped cranberries
1 cup (250 ml)	whole-wheat bread in small cubes
1	lightly beaten egg white
1/2 tsp.	salt
1/4 tsp.	pepper
1/4 tsp.	marjoram
1/4 tsp.	thyme
2	pork tenderloins 1 lb (500 g) each

- Heat oven to 325 °F (160 °C). Heat oil in a large non-stick frying pan. Add onion and celery, cook until soft but not yet brown. Add apple, currants, cranberries and bread cubes. Heat for 2 minutes, stirring. Remove from heat. Add egg white and seasonings, mix well, set aside.
- Remove all traces of fat from the tenderloins. Open them lengthwise, partway (as if you were opening a book). Place stuffing along the open side of one tenderloin. Close in a V and fold the other tenderloin above the opening. Tie with string so the two halves do not fall apart.
- Spray a non-stick frying pan with vegetable cooking spray and brown the rolled pork tenderloin on all sides.
- Place on the grill of a small roasting pan. Cover and cook for 1 1/2 hours. Cut the roll in slices and serve with orange sauce (see recipe, p. 211).

Pork tenderloin with dried fruit

6 SERVINGS

2/3 cup (160 ml)	dried apricots
5 tbsp.	raisins
2	pork tenderloins, 375 g (13 oz) each
1 tbsp.	olive oil
1	spanish onion
2	garlic cloves
2	carrots, cubed
1 cup (250 ml)	minced celery
1 cup (250 ml)	home-made chicken broth (see recipe, p. 113) or fat-free salt-free commercial broth
1 tbsp.	white wine vinegar
1/2 tsp. each	rosemary, marjoram, salt
1/4 tsp.	pepper
1 tbsp.	cornstarch
2 tbsp.	cold water

- Cover apricots and raisins with cold water and soak for 8 hours or overnight.
- Remove fat, slice the tenderloins. Brown slices in oil. Place in an ovenproof casserole.
- Brown onion, garlic, carrots and celery for 3 minutes over medium heat. Add broth, vinegar, rosemary, marjoram, salt and pepper. Bring to a boil. Pour over tenderloins. Cover and bake at 300 °F (150 °C) for 1 hour.
- Add drained apricots and raisins. Bake another 30 minutes.
- Just before serving, thicken cooking juices with cornstarch dissolved in cold water. Serve with basmati rice.

NUTRITIONAL VALUE PER SERVING

	Amount	% DV
Calories	270	
Fat	6 g	9%
Saturated	1.5 g	8%
+ Trans	0 g	
Polyunsaturated	0.5 g	
Omega-6	0.6 g	
Omega-3 (ALA)	0 g	
Omega-3 (EPA+DHA)	0 g	
Monounsaturated	3 g	
Cholesterol	74 mg	25%
Sodium	312 mg	13%
Potassium	918 mg	27%
Carbohydrate	23 g	8%
Dietary Fibre	3 g	13%
Sugars	16 g	
Protein	32 g	
Vitamin A		20%
Vitamin C		11%
Calcium		5%
Iron		19%
Vitamin D		3%
Vitamin E		13%

DIABETIC EXCHANGE

2 vegetables & fruits exchange
3 1/2 meat & alternatives exchanges
1/2 oils & fats exchange

Pork tenderloin with apples

4 SERVINGS

1	pork tenderloin, about 1 lb (500 g)
2 tbsp.	flour
1 tbsp.	olive oil
2	finely chopped green onions
1 cup (250 ml)	home-made beef broth (see recipe, p. 112) or fat-free salt-free commercial broth
2	cooking apples (Spartan or Cortland)
1/2 tsp.	salt
	Pepper to taste

- Cut tenderloin into 1 cm (1/2 inch) thick slices. Flatten them with a meat tenderizer or the edge of a saucer. Lightly flour.
- In a large non-stick frying pan, heat the oil and brown the loin slices. Add green onions and half the beef broth. Cook covered over low heat for 10 minutes. Add remaining beef broth, turn the meat slices over, add apples, which have been peeled and cut into 8 sections. Cook for another 10 minutes. Season. Serve the slices of meat garnished with pieces of apple.

Ham-tomato mousse

8 SERVINGS

2 envelopes	flavourless gelatine
300 ml (1 1/4 cup)	water
300 ml (1 1/4 cup)	tomato sauce (see recipe, p. 212)
1/2 cup (125 ml)	low-fat cottage cheese
2 tbsp.	lemon juice
1 tbsp.	onion, chopped very fine
1/2 cup (125 ml)	light mayonnaise
2 tsp.	Dijon mustard
2 cups (500 ml)	chopped cooked ham

- Soak gelatine in 1/4 cup (60 ml) water. Set aside.
- Mix the tomato sauce and remaining cup (250 ml) of water. Heat until boiling point. Remove from heat. Add gelatine and cottage cheese, combine well. Refrigerate. Add lemon juice, onion and mayonnaise, mustard and ham. Combine all ingredients.
- Apply non-stick vegetable spray to a ring-shaped jelly mould 8 inches (20 cm) in diameter. Pour in the ham mixture. Refrigerate until firm. Unmould onto a bed of lettuce.

NUTRITIONAL VALUE PER SERVING

	Amount	% DV
Calories	130	
Fat	7 g	12%
Saturated	1.5 g	8%
+ Trans	0 g	
Polyunsaturated	3.5 g	
Omega-6	2.9 g	
Omega-3 (ALA)	0.3 g	
Omega-3 (EPA+DHA)	0 g	
Monounsaturated	2 g	
Cholesterol	21 mg	7%
Sodium	670 mg	28%
Potassium	274 mg	8%
Carbohydrate	5 g	2%
Dietary Fibre	0.5 g	3%
Sugars	3 g	
Protein	10 g	
Vitamin A		1%
Vitamin C		12%
Calcium		2%
Iron		7%
Vitamin D		2%
Vitamin E		18%

DIABETIC EXCHANGE

2 meat & alternatives exchanges
1 oils & fats exchange

Roast pork with herbs
8 SERVINGS

NUTRITIONAL VALUE PER SERVING

	Amount	% DV
Calories	290	
Fat	13 g	20%
Saturated	4.5 g	22%
+ Trans	0 g	
Polyunsaturated	1.5 g	
Omega-6	1.2 g	
Omega-3 (ALA)	0.1 g	
Omega-3 (EPA+DHA)	0 g	
Monounsaturated	6.5 g	
Cholesterol	122 mg	41%
Sodium	382 mg	16%
Potassium	738 mg	22%
Carbohydrate	5 g	2%
Dietary Fibre	0.5 g	2%
Sugars	2 g	
Protein	38 g	
Vitamin A		2%
Vitamin C		22%
Calcium		3%
Iron		20%
Vitamin D		8%
Vitamin E		7%

DIABETIC EXCHANGE

5 meat & alternatives exchanges

1	boned pork roast of 3 lb (1.5 kg)

MARINADE:

2	chopped dried shallots
3	garlic cloves
3	sliced green onions
1/2 cup (125 ml)	fresh-squeezed orange juice
1 tbsp.	low-sodium soya sauce
1 tbsp.	olive oil
2 tsp.	balsamic vinegar
1 tsp.	ground cloves
1/2 tsp.	rosemary
1/2 tsp.	marjoram
1/2 tsp.	sage
1/2 tsp.	salt
1/4 tsp.	pepper
1/4 tsp.	curry

- Trim the meat, removing visible fat. Set the meat aside. Pour all other ingredients into the blender to make the marinade.
- Place the roast in a thick plastic bag. Add marinade. Expel the air from the bag and carefully seal. Place in a big bowl and refrigerate for 6 hours. Remove from refrigerator 30 minutes before cooking.
- Heat oven to 325 °F (160 °C). Place the roast on the grill in a roasting pan. Sprinkle with half the marinade. Cover and bake for 3 to 3 1/2 hours, or until meat is well done. Baste hourly with the cooking juices. Add remaining marinade if necessary. Carve and serve.

Veal chops provençale

4 SERVINGS

<table>
<tr><td>4</td><td>ripe tomatoes</td></tr>
<tr><td>1 tbsp.</td><td>olive oil</td></tr>
<tr><td>1</td><td>small chopped green onion</td></tr>
<tr><td>1</td><td>chopped dried shallot</td></tr>
<tr><td>2</td><td>chopped garlic cloves</td></tr>
<tr><td>1/4 tsp.</td><td>thyme</td></tr>
<tr><td>1 tsp.</td><td>sage</td></tr>
<tr><td>1</td><td>small celery stalk with leaves, whole</td></tr>
<tr><td>1/2 tsp.</td><td>salt</td></tr>
<tr><td></td><td>Pepper to taste</td></tr>
<tr><td>1 tbsp.</td><td>chopped parsley</td></tr>
<tr><td>4</td><td>good-sized veal chops, fat removed</td></tr>
<tr><td>12</td><td>pitted black olives, rinsed</td></tr>
</table>

- Blanch tomatoes in boiling water for a few seconds, cool, peel and chop.
- Heat oil in a medium-sized saucepan. Brown the green onion, shallot and garlic. Cook over low heat for 2 minutes, stirring. Add tomatoes, thyme, sage, celery stalk, salt and pepper. Cook uncovered over low heat for 45 to 60 minutes, stirring occasionally.
- Lightly oil a cast-iron frying pan with a ribbed bottom, brown chops over high heat for 2 minutes per side. Reduce heat, cook on low for 6 minutes per side.
- Remove celery stalk from tomato sauce. Add black olives. Serve sauce with the veal chops.
- Garnish with a bit of chopped parsley.

NUTRITIONAL VALUE PER SERVING

	Amount	% DV
Calories	270	
Fat	10 g	16%
Saturated	2.5 g	14%
+ Trans	0.1 g	
Polyunsaturated	1.5 g	
Omega-6	1.1 g	
Omega-3 (ALA)	0.1 g	
Omega-3 (EPA+DHA)	0 g	
Monounsaturated	5.5 g	
Cholesterol	106 mg	36%
Sodium	588 mg	25%
Potassium	857 mg	25%
Carbohydrate	10 g	4%
Dietary Fibre	2.5 g	10%
Sugars	1 g	
Protein	36 g	
Vitamin A		6%
Vitamin C		29%
Calcium		6%
Iron		24%
Vitamin D		74%
Vitamin E		16%

DIABETIC EXCHANGE

3 meat & alternatives exchanges
1 oils & fats exchange
1 vegetables & fruits exchange

Cubed veal with paprika

6 SERVINGS

1 1/2 lb (750 g)	boned veal shoulder
1 tbsp.	olive oil
2	large onions, minced
1/2 tsp.	salt
	Pepper to taste
1/4 tsp.	rosemary
1/4 tsp.	tarragon
2 tsp.	paprika
3/4 cup (180 ml)	half dry white wine-half chicken broth, home-made or store-bought (see recipe p. 113)
1 cup (250 ml)	diced carrots
1 cup (250 ml)	sliced mushrooms

- Thoroughly remove fat from meat and cut into 1 inch (2.5 cm) cubes.
- In a large non-stick frying pan, heat oil and brown the onions. Remove from the pan and set aside for later use.
- Lightly brown the veal cubes in the frying pan for about 10 minutes.
- Transfer meat to a non-stick saucepan. Add salt, pepper, rosemary and tarragon. Cook 10 minutes at medium-low.
- Add onions and paprika, combine over heat for 2 or 3 minutes. Add white wine, chicken broth and carrots. Cook on low for 30 minutes. Add mushrooms and cook another 15 minutes, or until meat is tender.
- Serve hot.

NUTRITIONAL VALUE PER SERVING

	Amount	% DV
Calories	205	
Fat	6 g	9%
Saturated	1.5 g	7%
+ Trans	0 g	
Polyunsaturated	0.5 g	
Omega-6	0.6 g	
Omega-3 (ALA)	0 g	
Omega-3 (EPA+DHA)	0 g	
Monounsaturated	2.5 g	
Cholesterol	105 mg	35%
Sodium	325 mg	14%
Potassium	636 mg	19%
Carbohydrate	9 g	3%
Dietary Fibre	1.5 g	7%
Sugars	4 g	
Protein	27 g	
Vitamin A		15%
Vitamin C		9%
Calcium		4%
Iron		12%
Vitamin D		53%
Vitamin E		11%

DIABETIC EXCHANGE

3 meat & alternatives exchanges
1 oils & fats exchange
1 vegetables & fruits exchange

Veal galantine

8 SERVINGS (MAIN COURSE) OR

2	veal shanks, about 3 lb (1.5 kg) total
1	large chopped onion
1/2 tsp.	rosemary
1/2 tsp.	basil
1	bay leaf
1 tsp.	salt
1 tbsp.	chopped parsley
1/4 tsp.	peppercorns
1	celery stalk with leaves
1	sliced carrot

- Place all ingredients in a large saucepan with lid. Add cold water to cover. Bring to a boil. Reduce heat and simmer on low for 2 hours.
- Cool broth, skim off fat and strain. Remove meat from the broth, remove bone. Chop veal finely. Reheat broth and add meat.
- Place in a mould cooled down with cold water, then oiled.
- Allow to set in the refrigerator. Unmould and decorate according to taste.

NUTRITIONAL VALUE PER SERVING

	Amount	% DV
Calories	190	
Fat	3 g	5%
Saturated	1 g	5%
+ Trans	0 g	
Polyunsaturated	0.5 g	
Omega-6	0.4 g	
Omega-3 (ALA)	0 g	
Omega-3 (EPA+DHA)	0 g	
Monounsaturated	1 g	
Cholesterol	168 mg	56%
Sodium	494 mg	21%
Potassium	698 mg	20%
Carbohydrate	3 g	2%
Dietary Fibre	0.5 g	3%
Sugars	1 g	
Protein	36 g	
Vitamin A		7%
Vitamin C		5%
Calcium		5%
Iron		27%
Vitamin D		38%
Vitamin E		1%

DIABETIC EXCHANGE

3 meat & alternatives exchanges
1/2 vegetables & fruits exchange

Osso bucco milanaise

4 SERVINGS

NUTRITIONAL VALUE PER SERVING

	Amount	% DV
Calories	340	
Fat	7 g	11%
Saturated	1.5 g	8%
+ Trans	0 g	
Polyunsaturated	1.5 g	
Omega-6	0.9 g	
Omega-3 (ALA)	0.1 g	
Omega-3 (EPA+DHA)	0 g	
Monounsaturated	3.5 g	
Cholesterol	201 mg	67%
Sodium	733 mg	31%
Potassium	1248 mg	36%
Carbohydrate	18 g	6%
Dietary Fibre	3 g	13%
Sugars	9 g	
Protein	46 g	
Vitamin A		21%
Vitamin C		23%
Calcium		11%
Iron		41%
Vitamin D		45%
Vitamin E		14%

DIABETIC EXCHANGE

2 vegetables & fruits exchanges
4 meat & alternatives exchanges
1/2 oils & fats exchange

1 tbsp.	olive oil
4	veal shanks, 1 1/2 inches (4 cm) thick, 1/2 lb (225 g) each
2	large onions cut in rings
2	garlic cloves
1 cup (250 ml)	carrots cut in rounds
1 cup (250 ml)	sliced celery
1/2 cup (125 ml)	dry white wine
180 ml (3/4 cup)	home-made chicken broth (see recipe, p. 113) or fat-free salt-free commercial broth
1 cup (250 ml)	crushed canned tomatoes, drained
1/2 tsp.	salt
1/2 tsp.	*herbes de Provence* (see recipe, p. 259)
	Pepper to taste

- Heat oil in a large non-stick frying pan. Brown the shank slices on both sides. Place in a saucepan with a lid.
- In the same frying pan, cook onions, garlic, carrots and celery at medium heat for 8 to 10 minutes. Pour over shank slices. Add wine, chicken broth, crushed tomatoes and seasonings. Cover and allow to simmer for 1 1/2 hours or until meat is well cooked. Serve on a bed of rice with sauce poured over top.

Orange veal roast

6 SERVINGS

3 lb (1.5 kg)	grain-fed veal loin roast
1 tbsp.	olive oil
1	bay leaf
2	chopped onions
1 cup (250 ml)	juice of one orange and water
	Zest of one orange
15	crushed juniper berries
1 tsp.	salt
1/4 tsp.	pepper

- Remove all visible fat from the roast. Heat the oil in a large non-stick frying pan. Brown meat on all sides. Place in an ovenproof casserole and add all other ingredients. Cover.
- Bake at 325 °F (160 °C) for about 2 1/2 hours or until meat is tender.

NUTRITIONAL VALUE PER SERVING

	Amount	% DV
Calories	320	
Fat	6 g	10%
Saturated	2 g	9%
+ Trans	0 g	
Polyunsaturated	1 g	
Omega-6	0.6 g	
Omega-3 (ALA)	0.1 g	
Omega-3 (EPA+DHA)	0 g	
Monounsaturated	3 g	
Cholesterol	193 mg	65%
Sodium	565 mg	24%
Potassium	1068 mg	31%
Carbohydrate	8 g	3%
Dietary Fibre	1.5 g	7%
Sugars	3 g	
Protein	54 g	
Vitamin A		1%
Vitamin C		28%
Calcium		7%
Iron		26%
Vitamin D		55%
Vitamin E		4%

DIABETIC EXCHANGE

1/2 vegetables & fruits exchange
6 meat & alternatives exchanges
1/2 oils & fats exchange

Veal Marengo

6 SERVINGS

	Amount	% DV
NUTRITIONAL VALUE PER SERVING		
Calories	270	
Fat	7.5 g	12%
Saturated	2 g	9%
+ Trans	0 g	
Polyunsaturated	1 g	
Omega-6	0.8 g	
Omega-3 (ALA)	0.1 g	
Omega-3 (EPA+DHA)	0 g	
Monounsaturated	4 g	
Cholesterol	140 mg	47%
Sodium	621 mg	26%
Potassium	944 mg	27%
Carbohydrate	13 g	5%
Dietary Fibre	2.5 g	10%
Sugars	4 g	
Protein	37 g	
Vitamin A		4%
Vitamin C		23%
Calcium		6%
Iron		19%
Vitamin D		71%
Vitamin E		14%

DIABETIC EXCHANGE

1 vegetables & fruits exchange
6 meat & alternatives exchanges
1/2 oils & fats exchange

1 tbsp.	olive oil
2 lb (1 kg)	cubed veal, fat removed
4	small onions, cut in quarters
375 ml (1 1/2 cup)	sliced fresh mushrooms
1/2 cup (125 ml)	sliced celery
1 tbsp.	all-purpose flour
1/2 cup (125 ml)	home-made chicken broth (see recipe, p. 113) or fat-free salt-free commercial broth
3	tomatoes, blanched, peeled and chopped
2	chopped garlic cloves
1/3 cup (80 ml)	black olives, rinsed
1/4 cup (60 ml)	dry white wine
2 tbsp.	tomato paste
1 1/2 tsp.	chopped fresh thyme
1	bay leaf
1 tsp.	salt
1/4 tsp.	pepper
2 tbsp.	chopped fresh parsley

- Heat the oil in a large non-stick frying pan. Brown the veal cubes. Remove from pan, set aside.
- In the same pan, cook onions, mushrooms and celery at medium heat until onions are transparent.
- Add flour and cook 1 minute, stirring. Add chicken broth, tomatoes, garlic and olives. Combine well. Add veal cubes. Cover and simmer for 20 minutes.
- Add white wine, tomato paste and seasonings. Cover and allow to simmer on low heat for 1 hour. Sprinkle with parsley and serve on a bed of hot rice.

Avocados stuffed with chicken

4 SERVINGS

NUTRITIONAL VALUE PER SERVING		
	Amount	% DV
Calories	320	
Fat	24 g	37%
Saturated	3 g	17%
+ Trans	0 g	
Polyunsaturated	5 g	
Omega-6	4.7 g	
Omega-3 (ALA)	0.4 g	
Omega-3 (EPA+DHA)	0 g	
Monounsaturated	14 g	
Cholesterol	38 mg	13%
Sodium	219 mg	10%
Potassium	768 mg	22%
Carbohydrate	13 g	5%
Dietary Fibre	8 g	32%
Sugars	2 g	
Protein	18 g	
Vitamin A		4%
Vitamin C		62%
Calcium		4%
Iron		9%
Vitamin D		1%
Vitamin E		29%

1	small cooked skinless chicken breast
1	stalk chopped celery
2	chopped green onions
1/4	red pepper cut in little cubes
12	finely chopped pecans
2 tbsp.	light mayonnaise
2 tbsp.	plain fat-free yogourt
1/4 tsp.	salt
	Pepper to taste
1/4 tsp.	rosemary
2	ripe avocados
2 tbsp.	lemon juice

- Dice the chicken breast. Add celery, green onion, pepper and pecans. Set aside.
- Combine mayonnaise, yogourt, salt, pepper and rosemary. Set aside.
- Cut both avocados in half and remove the stone. Scoop out the flesh without breaking the skin. Dice flesh and sprinkle with lemon juice.
- Prepare the chicken and mayonnaise mixture. Gently add the cubes of avocado. Fill each half-shell until heaped with filling, and serve immediately.

Note Lemon juice or vinegar should be sprinkled on avocados to prevent them from turning brown on contact with air.

DIABETIC EXCHANGE
1/2 vegetables & fruits exchange
1 meat & alternatives exchange
4 oils & fats exchanges

Turkey scallopini with rosemary

4 SERVINGS

NUTRITIONAL VALUE
PER SERVING

	Amount	% DV
Calories	235	
Fat	4.5 g	7%
Saturated	1 g	6%
+ Trans	0 g	
Polyunsaturated	1 g	
Omega-6	0.5 g	
Omega-3 (ALA)	0.1 g	
Omega-3 (EPA+DHA)	0 g	
Monounsaturated	2.5 g	
Cholesterol	81 mg	27%
Sodium	238 mg	10%
Potassium	640 mg	19%
Carbohydrate	14 g	5%
Dietary Fibre	1.5 g	6%
Sugars	4 g	
Protein	34 g	
Vitamin A		2%
Vitamin C		17%
Calcium		6%
Iron		19%
Vitamin D		6%
Vitamin E		17%

DIABETIC EXCHANGE

3 meat & alternatives exchanges
1/2 oils & fats exchange
1/2 grain product exchange

4	large turkey breasts
1/4	tsp. salt
	Pepper to taste
1/4 tsp.	garlic powder
1/3 cup (80 ml)	flour
2 tsp.	olive oil
1 cup (250 ml)	home-made tomato sauce (see recipe, p. 212)
1/4 cup (60 ml)	dry white wine
1/2 tsp.	dried rosemary or 1 tbsp. fresh chopped rosemary
2 tbsp.	freshly grated parmesan
1 tbsp.	chopped fresh parsley

- Place the turkey pieces between two sheets of waxed paper and pound them with a mallet until they are 1/4 inch (0.5 cm) thick. Season with salt, pepper and garlic powder. Sprinkle with flour. Shake to remove excess.
- In a large non-stick frying pan, heat oil at medium heat and fry the scallopinis about 4 minutes per side, or until golden. Remove from pan and keep warm.
- At medium heat, combine tomato sauce, wine and rosemary. Cook, stirring, until the sauce is reduced by half.
- Remove from heat. Pour over scallopinis, sprinkle with freshly-grated parmesan and put under the grill for 2 minutes.
- Sprinkle with parsley and serve immediately.

Turkey brochettes

4 SERVINGS

(TRADITIONAL, MICROWAVE OR BARBECUE METHOD)

NUTRITIONAL VALUE PER SERVING

	Amount	% DV
Calories	235	
Fat	4 g	7%
Saturated	0.5 g	4%
+ Trans	0 g	
Polyunsaturated	0.5 g	
Omega-6	0.5 g	
Omega-3 (ALA)	0.1 g	
Omega-3 (EPA+DHA)	0 g	
Monounsaturated	2.5 g	
Cholesterol	61 mg	21%
Sodium	128 mg	6%
Potassium	585 mg	17%
Carbohydrate	23 g	8%
Dietary Fibre	1 g	5%
Sugars	20 g	
Protein	25 g	
Vitamin A		3%
Vitamin C		142%
Calcium		4%
Iron		13%
Vitamin D		9%
Vitamin E		9%

DIABETIC EXCHANGE

1 vegetables & fruits exchange
3 meat & alternatives exchanges
1/2 oils & fats exchange

MARINADE:

1 cup (250 ml)	sugar-free apple juice
1/2 cup (125 ml)	sugar-free pineapple juice
2	chopped garlic cloves
2 tbsp.	light soya sauce
1/4 cup (60 ml)	olive oil

1/2	small turkey breast, de-boned and cut in 1 1/2 inch (4 cm) pieces
	Red and green pepper, onions, mushrooms and big chunks of fresh or sugar-free canned pineapple

SAUCE:

1 1/2 cups (375 ml)	sugar-free pineapple juice
2 tsp.	cornstarch

- Combine marinade ingredients. Add turkey cubes and allow to marinate for at least 2 hours at room temperature.
- Prepare vegetables in individual servings and blanch in boiling water 1 minute.
- Drain the turkey cubes and slide onto brochette skewers, alternating with vegetables and pineapple chunks.

Brochettes can be cooked in 3 ways:
- 25 minutes in a traditional oven preheated to 400 °F (200 °C), turning the brochettes halfway through the cooking time;
- in the microwave, place 4 brochettes on the bacon grill (use bamboo skewers). Cook at medium intensity (7) for 13 to 15 minutes, turning and changing their position halfway through cooking time. Let sit for 5 minutes before serving.
- on the barbecue at medium-low heat, place brochettes on a grill 4 inches (10 cm) from the heat source. Cook for about 10 minutes per side (20 minutes in all).

Sauce:
- Heat pineapple juice and thicken with a touch of cornstarch. If there are any pineapple chunks left, they can be finely chopped and added to the sauce. Serve on a bed of white rice with chives or green onions and a green salad.
- If you wish, chicken breasts may be substituted for turkey.

Barbecued chicken breasts

4 SERVINGS

(COOKED ON THE BARBECUE)

NUTRITIONAL VALUE PER SERVING		
	Amount	% DV
Calories	300	
Fat	12 g	19%
Saturated	2 g	11%
+ Trans	0 g	
Polyunsaturated	2.5 g	
Omega-6	2.1 g	
Omega-3 (ALA)	0.1 g	
Omega-3 (EPA+DHA)	0 g	
Monounsaturated	7 g	
Cholesterol	116 mg	39%
Sodium	561 mg	24%
Potassium	595 mg	17%
Carbohydrate	2 g	1%
Dietary Fibre	0 g	1%
Sugars	1 g	
Protein	46 g	
Vitamin A		2%
Vitamin C		7%
Calcium		3%
Iron		9%
Vitamin D		12%
Vitamin E		13%

DIABETIC EXCHANGE
3 1/2 meat & alternatives exchanges 1 oils & fats exchange

MARINADE:

1/4 cup (60 ml)	olive oil
	Juice of 2 limes
	Zest of 1 lime
2 tbsp.	low-sodium soya sauce
1 tbsp.	sesame oil
2	finely chopped garlic cloves
1 tsp.	fresh chopped rosemary or 1/2 tsp. dried rosemary
1/2 tsp.	salt
1/4 tsp.	pepper
1 tbsp.	sesame seeds

4	half chicken breasts, skinned with fat removed, 7 oz (200 g) each

- Combine marinade ingredients. Place chicken pieces on a platter and pour marinade over top. Cover and refrigerate the chicken pieces for at least 3 hours and up to 8 hours, turning occasionally.
- On a barbecue at medium heat, cook chicken breasts for 40 to 45 minutes, turning and basting occasionally. Serve with Sweet-and-sour sauce (see recipe, page 205).

Note Place a drip pan filled with water on the coals beneath the chicken. Make sure that at least 1 inch (2.5 cm) of water remains in the pan throughout cooking; this prevents the formation of flames.

Chicken breast roll-ups

4 SERVINGS

NUTRITIONAL VALUE PER SERVING

	Amount	% DV
Calories	375	
Fat	13 g	21%
Saturated	2.5 g	13%
+ Trans	0 g	
Polyunsaturated	2.5 g	
Omega-6	1.9 g	
Omega-3 (ALA)	0.2 g	
Omega-3 (EPA+DHA)	0 g	
Monounsaturated	8 g	
Cholesterol	116 mg	39%
Sodium	473 mg	20%
Potassium	870 mg	25%
Carbohydrate	14 g	5%
Dietary Fibre	2 g	9%
Sugars	3 g	
Protein	50 g	
Vitamin A		4%
Vitamin C		16%
Calcium		4%
Iron		17%
Vitamin D		20%
Vitamin E		19%

DIABETIC EXCHANGE

1/2 vegetables & fruits exchange
4 meat & alternatives exchanges
2 oils & fats exchanges

4	half chicken breasts, 7 oz (200 g) each, skinned with fat removed
2 tbsp.	olive oil
1	chopped dried shallot
2	chopped green onions
1 cup (250 ml)	thinly sliced mushrooms
1/4 cup (60 ml)	breadcrumbs
3 tbsp.	wheat germ
1 tbsp.	chopped fresh basil
1/4 cup (60 ml)	chopped hazelnuts
1/2 tsp.	salt
1 pinch	pepper
1/3 cup (80 ml)	home-made chicken broth (see recipe, p. 113) or fat-free salt-free commercial broth
1 tbsp.	chili sauce
1/2 cup (125 ml)	dry white wine

- Remove visible fat from the chicken breasts. Place between sheets of waxed paper and flatten until they are 1/2 inch (1 cm) thick.
- In a large non-stick frying pan, heat 1 tbsp. olive oil. Add shallot, green onion and mushrooms, and cook 3 minutes until they soften. Add breadcrumbs, wheat germ, basil, hazelnuts, salt and pepper. Bind with broth and chili sauce.
- Place a quarter of the mixture on each half-breast. Roll them up and spear with toothpicks.
- In a heavy non-stick frying pan, heat the other 1 tbsp. of olive oil. Brown the rolled chicken breasts. Add white wine. Lower heat to medium-low. Cover and cook 40 minutes. Turn the 'roll-ups' 2 or 3 times as they cook. If necessary, add broth. Remove toothpicks and cut each roll into 3 or 4 slices. Serve with Vegetable rice or Rice ring with fine herbs (see recipes, pp. 129 and 130).

Chicken cacciatore

6 SERVINGS

NUTRITIONAL VALUE PER SERVING

	Amount	% DV
Calories	300	
Fat	6 g	10%
Saturated	1 g	7%
+ Trans	0 g	
Polyunsaturated	1 g	
Omega-6	0.8 g	
Omega-3 (ALA)	0.1 g	
Omega-3 (EPA+DHA)	0 g	
Monounsaturated	2.5 g	
Cholesterol	116 mg	39%
Sodium	538 mg	23%
Potassium	1016 mg	30%
Carbohydrate	13 g	5%
Dietary Fibre	2.5 g	11%
Sugars	7 g	
Protein	47 g	
Vitamin A		16%
Vitamin C		37%
Calcium		6%
Iron		13%
Vitamin D		17%
Vitamin E		18%

DIABETIC EXCHANGE

1 1/2 vegetables & fruits exchange
3 1/2 meat & alternatives exchanges
1/2 oils & fats exchange

1 tbsp.	olive oil
6	half chicken breasts 7 oz (200 g) each, skinned, fat removed
1	large chopped onion
1 cup (250 ml)	carrots cut in rounds
2	sliced celery stalks
1	chopped garlic clove
1 tsp.	dried basil
1 tsp.	dried rosemary
19 oz (540 ml)	canned crushed tomatoes
1/2 cup (125 ml)	dry white wine
1/2 tsp.	salt
1 pinch	pepper
1 cup (250 ml)	sliced mushrooms
2 tbsp.	chopped fresh parsley

- Preheat oven to 325 °F (160 °C). Heat oil in a large non-stick frying pan. Brown chicken breasts on both sides. Set aside.
- In the same pan, sauté onion, carrots, celery and garlic. Sprinkle with basil and rosemary. Stir.
- Drain tomatoes, saving the juice. Add tomatoes to the vegetable mixture and cook for 8 minutes over medium heat. Add wine and tomato juice, allow to bubble for another 10 minutes.
- Transfer to a casserole and place chicken breasts on top of vegetables mixture. Season, cover and bake for 1/2 hour. Add mushrooms and bake for another 30 minutes. Arrange chicken pieces on a serving platter. Keep warm.
- Cook sauce and vegetables over high heat for 5 to 8 minutes and reduce. Add parsley. Pour sauce over the chicken breasts. Serve.

Crispy chicken with herbs and spices

6 SERVINGS

3	large chicken breasts
1/3 cup (80 ml)	plain low-fat yogourt
3 tbsp.	Dijon mustard
3/4 cup (180 ml)	whole-wheat breadcrumbs
1/4 tsp. of each	onion salt, celery seeds, tarragon, thyme, marjoram, basil, chervil, oregano, pepper.

- Remove skin and fat from the chicken breasts, and divide each in half (6 pieces total). Dry well.
- Combine yogourt and mustard. Set aside. In another bowl, combine breadcrumbs and all other ingredients.
- With a pastry brush, apply yogourt mixture to each piece of chicken, then roll them in the breadcrumb mixture.
- Arrange on a large baking sheet covered with aluminium foil.
- Bake at 350 °F (180 °C) 45 to 50 minutes, or until the chicken is well-cooked and a nice golden colour.

NUTRITIONAL VALUE PER SERVING

	Amount	% DV
Calories	220	
Fat	3.5 g	6%
Saturated	1 g	5%
+ Trans	0 g	
Polyunsaturated	1 g	
Omega-6	0.9 g	
Omega-3 (ALA)	0.1 g	
Omega-3 (EPA+DHA)	0 g	
Monounsaturated	1 g	
Cholesterol	79 mg	27%
Sodium	366 mg	16%
Potassium	452 mg	13%
Carbohydrate	12 g	4%
Dietary Fibre	0.5 g	3%
Sugars	2 g	
Protein	34 g	
Vitamin A		1%
Vitamin C		3%
Calcium		7%
Iron		10%
Vitamin D		8%
Vitamin E		2%

DIABETIC EXCHANGE

3 meat & alternatives exchanges
1/2 grain product exchange

Fruited chicken with sesame seeds

4 SERVINGS

NUTRITIONAL VALUE PER SERVING

	Amount	% DV
Calories	280	
Fat	7 g	12%
Saturated	1.5 g	8%
+ Trans	0 g	
Polyunsaturated	1.5 g	
Omega-6	1.3 g	
Omega-3 (ALA)	0.1 g	
Omega-3 (EPA+DHA)	0 g	
Monounsaturated	4 g	
Cholesterol	87 mg	29%
Sodium	253 mg	11%
Potassium	752 mg	22%
Carbohydrate	17 g	6%
Dietary Fibre	1.5 g	7%
Sugars	9 g	
Protein	38 g	
Vitamin A		7%
Vitamin C		160%
Calcium		5%
Iron		14%
Vitamin D		17%
Vitamin E		11%

DIABETIC EXCHANGE

1 1/2 vegetables & fruits exchange
4 meat & alternatives exchanges
1/2 oils & fats exchange

3 cups (750 ml)	chicken breast cut in cubes
1 cup (250 ml)	small pieces of canned pineapple
1 tbsp.	low-sodium soya sauce
1 tbsp.	chopped fresh ginger
1 tbsp.	olive oil
1/2	red pepper cut in fine strips
1/2	yellow pepper cut in fine strips
1 cup (250 ml)	sliced mushrooms
5	green onions chopped in 1 inch (2.5 cm) pieces
1	chopped garlic clove
1/2 cup (125 ml)	home-made chicken broth (see recipe, p. 113) or fat-free salt-free commercial broth
1 tbsp.	cornstarch
1 tbsp.	toasted sesame seeds

- Drain pineapple, setting aside 1/4 cup (60 ml) juice. Mix this juice with the soya sauce and ginger, then add chicken and marinate for 30 minutes.
- In a large non-stick frying pan, heat the oil. Drain chicken, set marinade aside. Brown chicken for 3 minutes then remove from pan.
- Stir-fry red and yellow peppers, mushrooms, green onions and garlic for 2 minutes. Add chicken and pineapple. Reheat for 3 minutes.
- Mix chicken broth, marinade and cornstarch. Add to the chicken-vegetable mix. Cool several minutes until it thickens. Sprinkle with sesame seeds. Serve.

Chicken-vegetable stir-fry

4 SERVINGS

2	chicken breasts
2 tbsp.	olive oil
1	large onion, cut in large chunks
3	chopped garlic cloves
1 tbsp.	chopped fresh ginger
2	celery stalks cut diagonally
1 cup (250 ml)	broccoli flowerets
1 cup (250 ml)	cauliflower flowerets
1/2	red pepper chopped
1/2	green pepper chopped
3/4 cup (180 ml)	home-made chicken broth (see recipe, p. 113) or fat-free salt-free commercial broth
1 tbsp.	cornstarch
1/4 cup (60 ml)	cold water
1 tbsp.	low-sodium soya sauce
	Pepper to taste
2 cups (500 ml)	hot cooked rice

- Prepare chicken breasts. Remove skin, fat and bone. Cut into small 3/4 inch (2 cm) cubes. In a large pan or wok, heat the oil and brown chicken cubes. Let cook for several minutes. Remove from pan and set aside.
- In the same pan or wok, lightly brown onion, garlic and ginger. Add all vegetables. Sauté for several minutes. Add chicken broth, cover, bring to a boil and let cook for 5 minutes. Vegetables should still be crunchy. Thicken the sauce with the mixture of cold water, cornstarch and soya sauce. Stir until sauce thickens. Season, add chicken and mix well.
- Serve on a bed of rice.

NUTRITIONAL VALUE PER SERVING

	Amount	% DV
Calories	350	
Fat	9.5 g	15%
Saturated	1.5 g	8%
+ Trans	0 g	
Polyunsaturated	1.5 g	
Omega-6	1.1 g	
Omega-3 (ALA)	0.2 g	
Omega-3 (EPA+DHA)	0 g	
Monounsaturated	6 g	
Cholesterol	58 mg	20%
Sodium	257 mg	11%
Potassium	718 mg	21%
Carbohydrate	37 g	13%
Dietary Fibre	3 g	12%
Sugars	5 g	
Protein	29 g	
Vitamin A		6%
Vitamin C		156%
Calcium		6%
Iron		11%
Vitamin D		6%
Vitamin E		19%

DIABETIC EXCHANGE

3 meat & alternatives exchanges
1 1/2 oils & fats exchange
1/2 vegetables & fruits exchange
1 grain product exchange

September chicken

4 SERVINGS

	Amount	% DV
NUTRITIONAL VALUE PER SERVING		
Calories	285	
ipides	9 g	14%
Saturated	2 g	10%
+ Trans	0.1g	
Polyunsaturated	1.5 g	
Omega-6	1.3 g	
Omega-3 (ALA)	0.1 g	
Omega-3 (EPA+DHA)	0.1 g	
Monounsaturated	4 g	
Cholesterol	104 mg	35%
Sodium	433 mg	19%
Potassium	564 mg	17%
Carbohydrate	25 g	9%
Dietary Fibre	2.5 g	11%
Sugars	20 g	
Protein	27 g	
Vitamin A		3%
Vitamin C		40%
Calcium		3%
Iron		13%
Vitamin D		3%
Vitamin E		12%

DIABETIC EXCHANGE

3 meat & alternatives exchanges
2 vegetables & fruits exchanges
1/2 oils & fats exchange
1 grain product exchange

4	whole chicken legs, skin removed

MARINADE:

2 cups (500 ml)	apple juice
1	bay leaf
1/4 tsp.	thyme
1 tbsp.	olive oil
1 cup (250 ml)	home-made chicken broth (see recipe, p. 113) or fat-free salt-free commercial broth
4	unpeeled cooking apples, cut in quarters
1/2 tsp.	salt
	Pepper to taste

- Marinate chicken pieces in refrigerator for at least 8 hours, in the apple juice combined with bay leaf, thyme, salt and pepper.
- Drain chicken and set marinade aside.
- In a large non-stick frying pan, at medium high, brown chicken on both sides in oil and margarine. Arrange in a casserole dish. Deglaze pan with marinade, and allow the liquid to reduce by half. Pour over chicken pieces. Add chicken broth and pieces of apple.
- Bake uncovered at 350 °F (180 °C) for 1 hour, or until chicken is tender.

Chicken with tomatoes

4 SERVINGS

2	big chicken breasts or 6 legs
1	chopped spanish onion
2	chopped garlic cloves
19 oz (540 ml)	canned stewed tomatoes with juice
1/2 tsp.	salt
1/2 tsp.	oregano
1/2 tsp.	basil
1 tbsp.	chopped fresh parsley
1/8 tsp.	pepper

- Prepare chicken. Remove skin and fat. Cut each breast into 4 pieces; legs may remain in one piece. In a large non-stick frying pan, brown chicken pieces on both sides.
- Mix vegetables and seasonings.
- Place chicken pieces in a heavy cooking pot and cover with vegetable mixture. Cover and cook at very low heat until meat is tender, between 1 and 1 1/4 hour.
- If you want to thicken the sauce, remove chicken pieces, increase heat and reduce sauce, stirring. Return chicken pieces to pot. Reheat for several minutes and serve.

NUTRITIONAL VALUE PER SERVING

	Amount	% DV
Calories	205	
Fat	2.5 g	4%
Saturated	1 g	5%
+ Trans	0 g	
Polyunsaturated	0.5 g	
Omega-6	0.4 g	
Omega-3 (ALA)	0.1 g	
Omega-3 (EPA+DHA)	0 g	
Monounsaturated	1 g	
Cholesterol	78 mg	26%
Sodium	672 mg	28%
Potassium	795 mg	23%
Carbohydrate	14 g	5%
Dietary Fibre	2.5 g	11%
Sugars	7 g	
Protein	32 g	
Vitamin A		3%
Vitamin C		44%
Calcium		5%
Iron		10%
Vitamin D		8%
Vitamin E		17%

DIABETIC EXCHANGE

3 meat & alternatives exchanges
1 1/2 vegetables & fruits exchange

Chicken fruit rolls

4 SERVINGS

NUTRITIONAL VALUE PER SERVING

	Amount	% DV
Calories	260	
Fat	6 g	9%
Saturated	1 g	6%
+ Trans	0 g	
Polyunsaturated	1 g	
Omega-6	0.7 g	
Omega-3 (ALA)	0.1 g	
Omega-3 (EPA+DHA)	0 g	
Monounsaturated	3 g	
Cholesterol	78 mg	26%
Sodium	609 mg	26%
Potassium	565 mg	17%
Carbohydrate	20 g	7%
Dietary Fibre	1.5 g	6%
Sugars	15 g	
Protein	31 g	
Vitamin A		2%
Vitamin C		32%
Calcium		3%
Iron		7%
Vitamin D		8%
Vitamin E		9%

DIABETIC EXCHANGE

3 meat & alternatives exchanges
1 vegetables & fruits exchange
1/2 oils & fats exchange

2	chicken breasts of about 3/4 lb (375 g) each

STUFFING:

1 tbsp.	finely chopped onion
1	finely chopped dried shallot
1 tbsp.	chopped fresh parsley
2 tbsp.	chopped celery
1/2 tsp.	well-crushed coriander seeds
1/8 tsp.	garlic powder
1 pinch	pepper
1 tbsp.	olive oil
1 cup (250 ml)	sugar-free pineapple chunks, set juice aside
1 cup (250 ml)	water
1/2 cup (125 ml)	sugar-free pineapple juice (from the chunks)
1 1/2 tbsp.	cornstarch
2 tbsp.	ketchup
1 tbsp.	low-sodium soya sauce
2 tsp.	wine or raspberry vinegar
1 tsp.	powdered chicken broth concentrate, without salt or fat
1/2 tsp.	salt
3/4 cup (180 ml)	mandarin orange sections

- Remove skin, fat and bones, ending up with 4 big pieces of chicken. Flatten between two sheets of wax paper, using a rolling pin, until they are about 1/4 inch (0.5 cm) thick.
- Mix stuffing ingredients and divide over each piece of chicken.
- Fold up the sides to keep the stuffing inside, and roll each like a jellyroll. Secure with oven skewers or string. Heat oil in a large non-stick frying pan. Brown chicken rolls on all sides. Add pineapple chunks. Set aside.
- In a small saucepan, mix all other ingredients except the mandarin oranges.
- Heat until sauce is a little thicker and translucent. Pour over chicken and cook on low for 30 to 40 minutes, or until chicken is thoroughly cooked and tender.
- Add mandarins 5 minutes before the end of cooking.

Blueberry chicken tournedos

4 SERVINGS

NUTRITIONAL VALUE PER SERVING		
	Amount	% DV
Calories	250	
Fat	8 g	13%
Saturated	2 g	9%
+ Trans	0 g	
Polyunsaturated	1.5 g	
Omega-6	1.3 g	
Omega-3 (ALA)	0.1 g	
Omega-3 (EPA+DHA)	0.1 g	
Monounsaturated	4 g	
Cholesterol	104 mg	35%
Sodium	409 mg	18%
Potassium	523 mg	15%
Carbohydrate	11 g	4%
Dietary Fibre	1.5 g	6%
Sugars	6 g	
Protein	33 g	
Vitamin A		4%
Vitamin C		15%
Calcium		3%
Iron		11%
Vitamin D		8%
Vitamin E		9%

1 tbsp.	olive oil
4	chicken tournedos, 5 oz (150 g) each
2	chopped dried shallots
1/2 tsp.	salt
1/4 tsp.	pepper
1 tbsp.	raspberry vinegar
1/2 cup (125 ml)	dry white wine
1 cup (250 ml)	fresh or frozen blueberries

- Heat oven to 350 °F (180 °C). Heat oil in a large non-stick frying pan. Brown tournedos on both sides. Add shallots and lightly brown. Add salt and pepper.
- Arrange tournedos in an ovenproof casserole, set aside.
- Deglaze the pan with raspberry vinegar and white wine for 2 minutes, add blueberries. Allow to simmer for 2 minutes, then pour over the tournedos. Bake for 45 minutes. If the sauce becomes too thick, add a bit of water. Serve the tournedos with the blueberry sauce.

DIABETIC EXCHANGE

1/2 vegetables & fruits exchange
4 meat & alternatives exchanges
1/2 oils & fats exchange

187

Fish and Seafood

Scallops on the half-shell

8 SERVINGS

**NUTRITIONAL VALUE
PER SERVING**

	Amount	% DV
Calories	210	
Fat	8 g	13%
Saturated	2 g	11%
+ Trans	0 g	
Polyunsaturated	1 g	
Omega-6	0.7 g	
Omega-3 (ALA)	0.1 g	
Omega-3 (EPA+DHA)	0.3 g	
Monounsaturated	4.5 g	
Cholesterol	50 mg	17%
Sodium	438 mg	19%
Potassium	425 mg	13%
Carbohydrate	9 g	3%
Dietary Fibre	0.5 g	2%
Sugars	3 g	
Protein	24 g	
Vitamin A		5%
Vitamin C		6%
Calcium		12%
Iron		8%
Vitamin D		18%
Vitamin E		12%

DIABETIC EXCHANGE

3 meat & alternatives exchanges
1 oils & fats exchange

8	coquille Saint-Jacques shells
1 lb (500 g)	small scallops
3/4 cup (180 ml)	water
1/2 tsp.	salt
	1% milk
3 tbsp.	olive oil
1 1/2 tbsp.	minced dried shallot
1 cup (250 ml)	fresh sliced mushrooms
2 tbsp.	flour
2 tsp.	lemon juice
1 cup (250 ml)	lobster or crab
7 oz (198 ml)	tuna canned in water, drained
1/3 cup (80 ml)	breadcrumbs
1/3 cup (80 ml)	light Emmenthal (15% M.F.)

- Put scallops in saucepan with water and salt. Simmer for 5 minutes. Drain. Keep the cooking liquid and add enough milk to make 1 1/2 cups (375 ml) of liquid. Set aside.
- At low heat, cook shallots and mushrooms in 1 tbsp. olive oil for 2 minutes, until golden. Set aside.
- In a medium-sized saucepan, melt remaining margarine, add flour and stir. Add liquid. Whisk over low heat until mixture thickens. Add lemon juice, shallot, mushrooms, scallops, lobster or crab, and tuna. Combine. Pour over coquille Saint-Jacques shells which have been sprayed with non-stick vegetable spray. Mix breadcrumbs and grated cheese. Sprinkle over the scallops. Bake at 375 °F (190 °C) for 20 to 30 minutes.

Note For a complete meal, form a ring of mashed potatoes and pour the fish mixture in the centre. The scallops can be prepared ahead of time. They just have to be covered with plastic wrap and frozen.

Plaice (sole) fillets provençale

4 SERVINGS

NUTRITIONAL VALUE PER SERVING		
	Amount	% DV
Calories	230	
Fat	10 g	15%
Saturated	1.5 g	8%
+ Trans	0 g	
Polyunsaturated	3 g	
Omega-6	2.4 g	
Omega-3 (ALA)	0.4 g	
Omega-3 (EPA+DHA)	0.3 g	
Monounsaturated	4 g	
Cholesterol	60 mg	20%
Sodium	393 mg	17%
Potassium	750 mg	22%
Carbohydrate	8 g	3%
Dietary Fibre	2 g	8%
Sugars	4 g	
Protein	25 g	
Vitamin A		5%
Vitamin C		119%
Calcium		5%
Iron		8%
Vitamin D		42%
Vitamin E		21%

DIABETIC EXCHANGE

3 meat & alternatives exchanges
1 vegetables & fruits exchange
1 oils & fats exchange

1	chopped spanish onion
1 tbsp.	olive oil
1 lb (500 g)	fresh plaice fillets
½ c. tsp.	salt
	Pepper to taste
½ tsp.	*herbes de Provence* (see recipe, p. 259)
½	chopped green pepper
½	chopped red pepper
6	large sliced mushrooms
2	chopped celery stalks
¼ cup (60 ml)	dry white wine
1 tbsp.	lemon juice

- Finely mince onion and arrange on the bottom of a flat 9-inch (22 cm) roasting pan. Dot with oil. Season the plaice fillets with salt, pepper and *herbes de Provence*. Place on top of the onions.
- Distribute vegetables evenly over the fish.
- Combine wine and lemon juice, and pour over top.
- Cook 25 to 30 minutes at 350 °F (180 °C) or until fish flakes easily with a fork.

Note Plaice is often confused with sole, which does not live in Canadian waters. Hence it is American plaice or winter flounder that often goes by the name "sole fillet" at the fish store.

Turbot fillets amandine

4 SERVINGS

1 lb (500 g)	turbot fillet
1/4 cup (60 ml)	all-purpose flour
1/2 tsp.	salt
1/4 cup (60 ml)	plain fat-free yogourt
1/4 cup (60 ml)	whole-wheat breadcrumbs
2 tbsp.	crushed almonds
2 tbsp.	chopped almonds
1/2 tbsp.	olive oil
1 tsp.	lemon juice

- Heat oven to 450 °F (230 °C). Separate fish into 4 individual servings. Coat these in flour and salt mixed together.
- With a pastry brush, dab yogourt on each piece of fish, then dip the pieces in breadcrumbs and crushed almonds mixed together.
- Place fish in a pyrex dish sprayed with non-stick vegetable spray. Bake for 15 minutes.
- Meanwhile, place chopped almonds in a small bowl. Add oil and cook in the microwave for 2 or 3 minutes at high intensity (10), or until they are golden. Stir once a minute. Add lemon juice. Sprinkle almonds on fillets. Serve.

NUTRITIONAL VALUE PER SERVING

	Amount	% DV
Calories	250	
Fat	9.5 g	15%
Saturated	1.5 g	9%
+ Trans	0 g	
Polyunsaturated	2.5 g	
Omega-6	1.3 g	
Omega-3 (ALA)	0.1 g	
Omega-3 (EPA+DHA)	1.1 g	
Monounsaturated	5 g	
Cholesterol	61 mg	21%
Sodium	547 mg	23%
Potassium	426 mg	13%
Carbohydrate	15 g	5%
Dietary Fibre	0.5 g	3%
Sugars	2 g	
Protein	25 g	
Vitamin A		2%
Vitamin C		5%
Calcium		8%
Iron		12%
Vitamin D		1%
Vitamin E		47%

DIABETIC EXCHANGE

1/2 grain product exchange
3 meat & alternatives exchanges
1/2 oils & fats exchange

Fish fillets with vegetables
4 SERVINGS

	Amount	% DV
NUTRITIONAL VALUE PER SERVING		
Calories	210	
Fat	5 g	8%
Saturated	1 g	4%
+ Trans	0 g	
Polyunsaturated	1 g	
Omega-6	0.6 g	
Omega-3 (ALA)	0.1 g	
Omega-3 (EPA+DHA)	0.2 g	
Monounsaturated	3 g	
Cholesterol	69 mg	23%
Sodium	476 mg	20%
Potassium	549 mg	16%
Carbohydrate	11 g	4%
Dietary Fibre	2 g	8%
Sugars	3 g	
Protein	31 g	
Vitamin A		5%
Vitamin C		46%
Calcium		6%
Iron		11%
Vitamin D		18%
Vitamin E		18%

DIABETIC EXCHANGE

3 meat & alternatives exchanges
1/2 vegetables & fruits exchange

1 tbsp.	olive oil
1	celery stalk, diced
1	small finely chopped onion
1	clove garlic, crushed
1/4 cup (60 ml)	yellow pepper, diced fine
1	diced fresh tomato
1 tsp.	*herbes de Provence* (see recipe, p. 259)
1/2 tsp.	salt
1/4 tsp.	pepper
1/4 cup (60 ml)	whole-wheat breadcrumbs
1 lb (500 g)	fillets of cod, haddock or turbot
2 tbsp.	chopped fresh parsley

- Heat oven to 450 °F (230 °C). Heat olive oil in a large non-stick frying pan. At medium heat, sauté celery, onion, garlic and pepper until tender. Add tomato, *herbes de Provence*, salt, pepper and breadcrumbs. Set aside.
- Apply non-stick vegetable spray to a pyrex dish. Divide fillets into individual portions. Arrange fillets in a single layer in the baking dish. Spread chopped vegetables over top. Bake 15 minutes. Sprinkle with chopped parsley and serve.

Fish fillets à l'orange

4 SERVINGS

NUTRITIONAL VALUE PER SERVING

	Amount	% DV
Calories	220	
Fat	7 g	13%
Saturated	1 g	6%
+ Trans	0 g	
Polyunsaturated	1 g	
Omega-6	0.7 g	
Omega-3 (ALA)	0.1 g	
Omega-3 (EPA+DHA)	0.2 g	
Monounsaturated	5 g	
Cholesterol	69 mg	23%
Sodium	397 mg	17%
Potassium	462 mg	14%
Carbohydrate	10 g	4%
Dietary Fibre	1 g	5%
Sugars	7 g	
Protein	30 g	
Vitamin A		4%
Vitamin C		58%
Calcium		4%
Iron		7%
Vitamin D		18%
Vitamin E		21%

DIABETIC EXCHANGE

3 meat & alternatives exchanges
1 oils & fats exchange
1/2 vegetables & fruits exchange

6 tbsp. (90 ml)	fresh orange juice
1	chopped onion
2 tbsp.	chopped parsley
1 tsp.	chopped fresh ginger
1/8 tsp.	cayenne pepper
2 tbsp.	canola, olive or peanut oil
1/2 tsp.	salt
	Pepper to taste
1 lb (500 g)	fillets of cod, halibut or haddock

GARNISHING:

1	orange, very finely sliced

- Prepare marinade: Mix orange juice, onion, parsley, ginger, cayenne pepper, oil, salt and pepper. Set aside.
- Prepare slices of fish, arrange in an ovenproof dish, sprinkle with marinade. Allow to marinate in the refrigerator for 2 hours.
- Heat oven to 350 °F (180 °C), bake fish 20 to 25 minutes. Serve garnished with thin slices of orange. Ladle cooking juices over top.

Trout fillets with fennel

4 SERVINGS

NUTRITIONAL VALUE PER SERVING

	Amount	% DV
Calories	205	
Fat	7 g	12%
Saturated	2.5 g	12%
+ Trans	0 g	
Polyunsaturated	2.5 g	
Omega-6	0.9 g	
Omega-3 (ALA)	0.1 g	
Omega-3 (EPA+DHA)	1.2 g	
Monounsaturated	2 g	
Cholesterol	77 mg	26%
Sodium	410 mg	18%
Potassium	627 mg	18%
Carbohydrate	2 g	1%
Dietary Fibre	0 g	1%
Sugars	1 g	
Protein	31 g	
Vitamin A		12%
Vitamin C		9%
Calcium		11%
Iron		4%
Vitamin D		1%
Vitamin E		1%

DIABETIC EXCHANGE

4 meat & alternatives exchanges

4	fillets rainbow trout 4.5 oz (125 g) each
1/4 tsp.	salt
1/4 tsp.	pepper
2 tbsp.	finely chopped chives

SAUCE:

1/2 cup (125 ml)	low-fat cottage cheese
2 tbsp.	plain fat-free yogourt
2 tbsp.	fresh chopped fennel
1/4 tsp.	salt
1/4 tsp.	pepper

- Heat oven to 400 °F (200 °C). Spray a big sheet of aluminium foil with non-stick vegetable spray. Arrange trout fillets on the foil in a single layer. Add salt and pepper, and sprinkle chives over top. Close the sheet of foil, sealing firmly. Place in a roasting pan and bake for 15 minutes.
- Put cottage cheese, yogourt, fennel, salt and pepper in a blender or food processor and mix for several seconds. Serve sauce with the fish.

Seafood-vegetable casserole

4 SERVINGS

NUTRITIONAL VALUE PER SERVING

	Amount	% DV
Calories	250	
Fat	7.5 g	14%
Saturated	1 g	6%
+ Trans	0 g	
Polyunsaturated	1.5 g	
Omega-6	0.8 g	
Omega-3 (ALA)	0.1 g	
Omega-3 (EPA+DHA)	0.3 g	
Monounsaturated	5 g	
Cholesterol	86 mg	29%
Sodium	684 mg	29%
Potassium	750 mg	22%
Carbohydrate	13 g	5%
Dietary Fibre	2 g	8%
Sugars	4 g	
Protein	32 g	
Vitamin A		22%
Vitamin C		107%
Calcium		8%
Iron		6%
Vitamin D		0%
Vitamin E		16%

DIABETIC EXCHANGE

3 meat & alternatives exchanges
1 oils & fats exchange
1 vegetables & fruits exchange

2 tbsp.	olive oil
1 lb (500 g)	scallops
1/2 lb (250 g)	crab or lobster meat, cut in cubes
2	minced celery stalks
1	minced carrot
1/2	green pepper cut in cubes
1/2	red pepper cut in cubes
1	finely chopped onion
	Pepper to taste
1/2 cup (125 ml)	home-made chicken broth (see recipe page 113) or fat-free salt-free commercial broth
2 tsp.	cornstarch
Thin slices	lemon to garnish

- Heat 1 tbsp. of the oil in a large non-stick frying pan. Add scallops, cook at medium heat for 2 minutes. Add crab or lobster and continue cooking for another 2 minutes, stirring constantly. Remove seafood from the pan and set aside.
- Add remaining oil to the frying pan. Add celery, carrots, green and red peppers, and onion. Cook 3 minutes, add chicken broth, reduce heat and simmer covered for 3 to 4 minutes. Season.
- Thicken sauce with cornstarch dissolved in 2 tbsp. cold water. Return seafood to the sauce. Mix and serve with rice flavoured with parsley, or on a bed of linguine.
- Garnish with lemon slices.

Mussels marinières

2 SERVINGS AS A MAIN COURSE

4 SERVINGS AS AN APPETIZER

2 lb (1 kg)	fresh mussels
1	small onion, chopped fine
1 tbsp.	chopped fresh parsley
1/4 tsp.	thyme
1/8 tsp.	garlic powder
	Pepper to taste
1/2 cup (125 ml)	dry white wine

- Wash the mussels with a stiff-bristled brush, discarding the ones that do not immediately open in cold water or if you hit them with your fingertips.
- Place all ingredients in a saucepan. Cover and cook at medium heat for 4 minutes. Stir mussels once or twice. Make sure all mussels are open.
- If necessary, cook for another 1 or 2 minutes. Throw out any mussels that still do not want to open.
- Serve with Fettuccine primavera (see recipe, p. 126) or whole wheat rusks.

Note In season, fresh mussels are not really expensive, and make an elegant and refined meal. They are low in fat and cholesterol.

NUTRITIONAL VALUE
PER SERVING (as an appetizer)

	Amount	% DV
Calories	125	
Fat	3 g	5%
Saturated	0.5 g	3%
+ Trans	0 g	
Polyunsaturated	1 g	
Omega-6	0 g	
Omega-3 (ALA)	0 g	
Omega-3 (EPA+DHA)	0.6 g	
Monounsaturated	0.5 g	
Cholesterol	35 mg	12%
Sodium	360 mg	15%
Potassium	446 mg	13%
Carbohydrate	7 g	3%
Dietary Fibre	0.5 g	2%
Sugars	1 g	
Protein	15 g	
Vitamin A		7%
Vitamin C		22%
Calcium		4%
Iron		37%
Vitamin D		4%
Vitamin E		7%

DIABETIC EXCHANGE

3 meat & alternatives exchanges
1/2 vegetables & fruits exchange

Crispy fish
4 SERVINGS

1 lb (500 g)	fillet of plaice (sole), turbot or cod
½ cup (125 ml)	1% milk
¼ tsp.	salt
¼ tsp.	pepper
1 cup (250 ml)	corn flakes, crumbled fine (Corn Flakes breakfast cereal)
2 tsp.	olive oil

- Divide fish into individual portions.
- Mix milk, salt and pepper. Dip the fish pieces in it, then roll them in the finely-crumbled cereal.
- Arrange in a lightly-oiled pyrex dish and drizzle fish pieces with remaining oil.
- Bake at 450 °F (230 °C) 15 minutes.

Note This fish goes very nicely with tomato coulis (see recipe, p. 202), garnished with fresh chopped chives.

NUTRITIONAL VALUE PER SERVING

	Amount	% DV
Calories	205	
Fat	4 g	7%
Saturated	1 g	5%
+ Trans	0 g	
Polyunsaturated	0.5 g	
Omega-6	0.2 g	
Omega-3 (ALA)	0 g	
Omega-3 (EPA+DHA)	0.3 g	
Monounsaturated	2 g	
Cholesterol	2 mg	21%
Sodium	343 mg	15%
Potassium	516 mg	15%
Carbohydrate	15 g	5%
Dietary Fibre	0.5 g	2%
Sugars	3 g	
Protein	26 g	
Vitamin A		4%
Vitamin C		4%
Calcium		6%
Iron		18%
Vitamin D		36%
Vitamin E		10%

DIABETIC EXCHANGE

3 meat & alternatives exchanges

Barbecued salmon

4 SERVINGS

(COOKED ON THE BARBECUE)

NUTRITIONAL VALUE PER SERVING		
	Amount	% DV
Calories	310	
Fat	20 g	31%
Saturated	3.5 g	19%
+ Trans	0 g	
Polyunsaturated	6 g	
Omega-6	1.2 g	
Omega-3 (ALA)	0.2 g	
Omega-3 (EPA+DHA)	2.9 g	
Monounsaturated	8.5 g	
Cholesterol	89 mg	30%
Sodium	90 mg	4%
Potassium	555 mg	16%
Carbohydrate	0 g	1%
Dietary Fibre	0 g	1%
Sugars	0 g	
Protein	30 g	
Vitamin A		3%
Vitamin C		11%
Calcium		2%
Iron		5%
Vitamin D		181%
Vitamin E		5%

DIABETIC EXCHANGE
4 meat & alternatives exchanges
2 oils & fats exchanges

4	salmon steaks, 5 oz (150 g) each

MARINADE:

1/4 cup (60 ml)	olive oil
1/4 cup (60 ml)	white wine
2 tbsp.	raspberry vinegar
2 tbsp.	chopped dried shallot
1	chopped garlic clove
1 tbsp.	chopped fresh dill

- Trim salmon steaks. Arrange in a single layer in a deep baking dish.
- Mix other ingredients and pour over the steaks. Cover and refrigerate at least 6 hours or better, overnight. Turn the steaks once or twice.
- Heat barbecue to medium heat. Spray non-stick vegetable spray on the grill.
- Drain the salmon steaks, set aside marinade. Grill steaks for 5 minutes on either side. Baste with marinade occasionally as they cook.

Seafood-stuffed tomatoes

6 SERVINGS

6	firm, good-sized tomatoes
1/2 cup (125 ml)	crab flesh
1/2 cup (125 ml)	scampi, cooked and cubed
1/2 cup (125 ml)	cooked fish (sole, haddock, trout, etc.)
2	green onions, finely chopped
1/2 cup (125 ml)	finely chopped celery
3 tbsp.	chopped red or green pepper
3/4 cup (180 ml)	tomato pulp
1/4 cup (60 ml)	light cholesterol-free salad dressing
1/4 tsp.	salt
	Pepper to taste

- Remove a slice from the bottom of each tomato. Extract pulp, drain in a colander for the stuffing.
- Once drained, add 3/4 cup (180 ml) of the pulp to the other ingredients. Stuff the tomatoes.
- Chill and decorate with parsley just before serving.

Note Seafood-stuffed tomatoes can also be served as a starter on a small lettuce leaf, or as part of a cold buffet.

NUTRITIONAL VALUE PER SERVING

	Amount	% DV
Calories	110	
Fat	4 g	6%
Saturated	0.5 g	4%
+ Trans	0 g	
Polyunsaturated	2.5 g	
Omega-6	2 g	
Omega-3 (ALA)	0.3 g	
Omega-3 (EPA+DHA)	0.2 g	
Monounsaturated	1 g	
Cholesterol	29 mg	10%
Sodium	296 mg	13%
Potassium	408 mg	12%
Carbohydrate	10 g	4%
Dietary Fibre	2 g	8%
Sugars	2 g	
Protein	10 g	
Vitamin A		6%
Vitamin C		36%
Calcium		3%
Iron		7%
Vitamin D		4%
Vitamin E		9%

DIABETIC EXCHANGE

1/2 meat & alternatives exchange
1 vegetables & fruits exchange
1/2 oils & fats exchange

Grilled trout papillotes

4 SERVINGS

(COOKED ON THE BARBECUE)

1 tbsp.	olive oil
1/2 cup (125 ml)	chopped celery
2/3 cup (160 ml)	grated carrots
3 tbsp.	chopped dried shallot
1 cup (250 ml)	croutons, crumbled
2 tbsp.	lemon juice
1/3 cup (80 ml)	dry white wine
1	whole trout, 2-3 lb (1-1.5 kg)
1/2 tsp.	salt
	Pepper to taste
1	thinly sliced lemon

- In a small frying pan heat oil and cook celery, carrots and shallot for 4 to 5 minutes at low heat.
- Mix with croutons and lemon juice. Moisten with white wine. Season trout and stuff. Secure with string.
- Generously oil the shiny side of a sheet of aluminium foil folded in two, big enough to fully envelop the fish. Brush the trout with oil.
- Place half the lemon slices on the sheet of foil. Lay the fish on them, then put the remaining lemon slices on top. Close the sheet of foil. Make sure the fold is fairly loose – the packet must be sealed well, but not tightly wrapped around the fish.
- The fish is cooked when the flesh is opaque.
- Place the fish in a large heated dish. Garnish with lemon slices and parsley sprigs.

Note The "papillote" cooking method is very well suited to whole fish such as trout, pike or walleye pike.

NUTRITIONAL VALUE PER SERVING

	Amount	% DV
Calories	210	
Fat	7.5 g	14%
Saturated	2 g	10%
+ Trans	0 g	
Polyunsaturated	1.5 g	
Omega-6	0.6 g	
Omega-3 (ALA)	0.1 g	
Omega-3 (EPA+DHA)	0.7 g	
Monounsaturated	4 g	
Cholesterol	104 mg	35%
Sodium	464 mg	20%
Potassium	600 mg	18%
Carbohydrate	12 g	4%
Dietary Fibre	1.5 g	7%
Sugars	2 g	
Protein	23 g	
Vitamin A		16%
Vitamin C		16%
Calcium		5%
Iron		8%
Vitamin D		176%
Vitamin E		7%

DIABETIC EXCHANGE

3 vegetables & fruits exchanges
4 meat & alternatives exchanges
1/2 oils & fats exchange

Fisherman's vol-au-vent

4 SERVINGS

NUTRITIONAL VALUE PER SERVING		
	Amount	% DV
Calories	315	
Fat	17 g	27%
Saturated	2.5 g	13%
+ Trans	0 g	
Polyunsaturated	2.5 g	
Omega-6	2.3 g	
Omega-3 (ALA)	0.2 g	
Omega-3 (EPA+DHA)	0.1 g	
Monounsaturated	11 g	
Cholesterol	39 mg	13%
Sodium	667 mg	28%
Potassium	431 mg	13%
Carbohydrate	25 g	9%
Dietary Fibre	3 g	13%
Sugars	7 g	
Protein	17 g	
Vitamin A		6%
Vitamin C		50%
Calcium		6%
Iron		17%
Vitamin D		5%
Vitamin E		25%

DIABETIC EXCHANGE

1/2 milk & alternatives exchange
1 grain product exchange
2 meat & alternatives exchanges
2 oils & fats exchanges

4 slices	whole wheat baguette
1 cup (250 ml)	small scallops
1/2 cup (125 ml)	water
	1% milk
1 tbsp.	olive oil
3	finely chopped green onions
1	finely chopped dried shallot
2/3 cup (160 ml)	sliced mushrooms
3 tbsp.	diced green pepper
3 tbsp.	diced red pepper
2 tbsp.	margarine
3 tbsp.	flour
1/2 cup (125 ml)	crab meat
1/2 tsp.	salt
	Pepper to taste
1/2 tsp.	oregano
4	good-sized shrimp
	Parsley for garnish

- Mould the bread slices into muffin moulds and place in an oven preheated to 350 °F (180 °C). Keep warm.
- Simmer the scallops in the water for 3 minutes. Drain and set aside cooking water. Add milk to obtain 375 ml (1 1/2 cup) of liquid. Set aside.
- Heat oil at low heat. Brown onions, shallot, mushrooms and the two peppers. Cook for 3 minutes. Set aside.
- In a medium-sized saucepan, melt the 2 tbsp. of margarine. Add flour, combining. Add the liquid, heat at low, whisking, until the mixture thickens. Add scallops, crab, and the vegetables. Season.
- Pour over the hot crusty bread, and garnish with a shrimp and a parsley sprig.

201
Sauces, Marinades
and Dips

Tomato coulis

MAKES 1 1/2 CUPS (375 ML)

NUTRITIONAL VALUE PER 1 TBSP. SERVING		
	Amount	% DV
Calories	15	
Fat	0.7 g	2%
Saturated	0.1 g	1%
+ Trans	0 g	
Polyunsaturated	0 g	
Omega-6	0.1 g	
Omega-3 (ALA)	0.1 g	
Omega-3 (EPA+DHA)	0 g	
Monounsaturated	0.5 g	
Cholesterol	0 mg	0%
Sodium	24 mg	1%
Potassium	85 mg	3%
Carbohydrate	2 g	1%
Dietary Fibre	0.5 g	3%
Sugars	1 g	
Protein	0.5 g	
Vitamin A		2%
Vitamin C		6%
Calcium		1%
Iron		2%
Vitamin D		0%
Vitamin E		2%

DIABETIC EXCHANGE
None

1 1/2 lb (750 g)	fresh tomatoes
1 tbsp.	olive oil
1	large chopped onion
1	clove of garlic
1	celery stalk with leaves
1/2 tsp.	basil
1/2 tsp.	tarragon
1/4 tsp.	oregano
1/4 tsp.	salt
1 pinch	pepper

- Blanch tomatoes 1 minute in boiling water. Allow to cool; peel and chop. Set aside.
- Heat the oil in a small saucepan. Cook onions, garlic and celery for 3 minutes at medium heat, until tender.
- Add tomatoes and remaining ingredients. Simmer half-covered at low heat for 15 minutes.
- Remove from heat and purée in the blender.

Note The coulis can also be made with canned tomatoes. In that case, use a 28 oz (796 ml) can of stewed tomatoes instead of fresh tomatoes. Proceed in the same way as above. This sauce freezes very well.

Orange marinade

MAKES 1 CUP (250 ML)

2	oranges
1 tbsp.	low-sodium soya sauce
1	chopped garlic clove
1	chopped dried shallot
1 tbsp.	chopped fresh ginger
1/4 cup (60 ml)	red wine
3 tbsp.	olive oil
1 pinch	pepper

- Zest the oranges. Extract the juice from both oranges. Combine all ingredients.
- Marinate meat for 2 to 6 hours, drain, and grill.

NUTRITIONAL VALUE PER 1 TBSP. SERVING

	Amount	% DV
Calories	33	
Fat	41 g	2.6%
Saturated	0.3 g	4%
+ Trans	0 g	
Polyunsaturated	0.2 g	
Omega-6	0.2 g	
Omega-3 (ALA)	0 g	
Omega-3 (EPA+DHA)	0 g	
Monounsaturated	1.9 g	
Cholesterol	0 mg	0%
Sodium	39 mg	2%
Potassium	40 mg	1%
Carbohydrate	2.2 g	1%
Dietary Fibre	0.2 g	1%
Sugars	1.1 g	
Protein	0.2 g	
Vitamin A		0%
Vitamin C		11%
Calcium		0%
Iron		1%
Vitamin D		0%
Vitamin E		4%

DIABETIC EXCHANGE

None

Pesto

MAKES 375 ML (1 ¹/2 CUP)

NUTRITIONAL VALUE PER 1 TBSP. SERVING		
	Amount	% DV
Calories	45	
Fat	4 g	7%
Saturated	0.5 g	4%
+ Trans	0 g	
Polyunsaturated	1 g	
Omega-6	0.8 g	
Omega-3 (ALA)	0.1 g	
Omega-3 (EPA+DHA)	0 g	
Monounsaturated	2.5 g	
Cholesterol	1 mg	1%
Sodium	18 mg	1%
Potassium	30 mg	1%
Carbohydrate	1 g	1%
Dietary Fibre	0 g	1%
Sugars	1 g	
Protein	1 g	
Vitamin A		2%
Vitamin C		7%
Calcium		2%
Iron		3%
Vitamin D		1%
Vitamin E		6%

DIABETIC EXCHANGE
1 oils & fats exchange

¹/2 cup (125 ml)	well-packed, fresh basil
¹/2 cup (125 ml)	well-packed, fresh parsley
2	large garlic cloves
¹/4 cup (60 ml)	pine nuts
¹/4 cup (60 ml)	grated parmesan
¹/3 cup (80 ml)	olive oil

- Remove basil and parsley leaves from their stems. Discard all stems. Rinse leaves and dry.
- In a food processor, combine parsley, basil, garlic, pine nuts, parmesan and 2 tbsp. olive oil.
- With a spatula, scrape down the sides of the food processor bowl. Start again, slowly adding the rest of the oil through the opening on top. Scrape the sides of the bowl a second time, and mix for another 2 to 3 seconds.

Note Pesto will keep 5 days in the refrigerator and about 3 months in the freezer.

Sweet-and-sour sauce

MAKES 1 1/2 CUPS (375 ML)

NUTRITIONAL VALUE
PER 1/4 CUP (60 ML) SERVING

	Amount	% DV
Calories	55	
Fat	0 g	0%
Saturated	0 g	0%
+ Trans	0 g	
Polyunsaturated	0 g	
Omega-6	0 g	
Omega-3 (ALA)	0 g	
Omega-3 (EPA+DHA)	0 g	
Monounsaturated	0 g	
Cholesterol	0 mg	0%
Sodium	260 mg	11%
Potassium	124 mg	4%
Carbohydrate	14 g	5%
Dietary Fibre	1 g	4%
Sugars	12 g	
Protein	1 g	
Vitamin A		1%
Vitamin C		13%
Calcium		2%
Iron		3%
Vitamin D		0%
Vitamin E		1%

DIABETIC EXCHANGE

1/2 vegetables & fruits exchange

14 oz (400 ml)	crushed unsweetened canned pineapple
2 tbsp.	low-sodium soya sauce
2 tbsp.	ketchup
1 tbsp.	cornstarch
3 tbsp.	white wine vinegar
2 tbsp.	low-calorie sweetener (Splenda)

- Bring to a boil the pineapple (undrained), soya sauce and ketchup.
- Dissolve the cornstarch in the wine vinegar, and add to preceding mixture.
- Reduce heat and let sauce simmer for 5 minutes, whisking. Remove from heat and add sweetener.
- Serve with chicken, turkey or pork tournedos.

Barbecue sauce
MAKES 1 1/2 CUPS (375 ML)

NUTRITIONAL VALUE PER 1 TBSP. SERVING

	Amount	% DV
Calories	12	
Fat	0.6 g	1%
Saturated	0.1 g	1%
+ Trans	0 g	
Polyunsaturated	0.2 g	
Omega-6	0.1 g	
Omega-3 (ALA)	0.1 g	
Omega-3 (EPA+DHA)	0 g	
Monounsaturated	0.4 g	
Cholesterol	0 mg	0%
Sodium	60 mg	3%
Potassium	59 mg	2%
Carbohydrate	1.5 g	1%
Dietary Fibre	0 g	1%
Sugars	1 g	
Protein	0.3 g	
Vitamin A		2%
Vitamin C		11%
Calcium		1%
Iron		2%
Vitamin D		0%
Vitamin E		2%

DIABETIC EXCHANGE
None

1 tbsp.	olive oil
1	chopped dried shallot
1	chopped garlic clove
2 cups (500 ml)	vegetable juice
1 tbsp.	tomato paste
1 tsp.	Dijon mustard
2 tbsp.	tarragon wine vinegar
	A few drops of tabasco sauce
1 pinch	pepper
1/4 tsp.	paprika
1/4 tsp.	oregano
1 tsp.	chopped parsley

- In a heavy pot, cook shallot at medium heat for 2 to 3 minutes in the oil. Add garlic, cook for 1 minute. Add juice and tomato paste, mustard, vinegar and tabasco sauce. Season with the remaining ingredients.

- Simmer on low for 30 minutes. Half-cover the pot. The sauce will thicken as it cools. Keep in refrigerator.

Note This sauce is delicious on barbecued steak or oven-baked chicken, such as Crispy chicken with herbs and spices (see recipe, p. 179)

Lemon sauce
MAKES 1 1/4 CUPS (300 ML)

NUTRITIONAL VALUE PER 1 TBSP. SERVING

	Amount	% DV
Calories	5	
Fat	0.1 g	0%
Saturated	0 g	0%
+ Trans	0 g	
Polyunsaturated	0 g	
Omega-6	0 g	
Omega-3 (ALA)	0 g	
Omega-3 (EPA+DHA)	0 g	
Monounsaturated	0 g	
Cholesterol	0 mg	0%
Sodium	30 mg	2%
Potassium	18 mg	1%
Carbohydrate	0.5 g	1%
Dietary Fibre	0 g	1%
Sugars	1 g	
Protein	0.5 g	
Vitamin A		1%
Vitamin C		1%
Calcium		1%
Iron		1%
Vitamin D		0%
Vitamin E		1%

DIABETIC EXCHANGE
None

1 1/2 cups (375 ml)	home-made chicken broth (see recipe p. 113) or fat-free salt-free commercial brand
1 tbsp.	lemon juice
2 tsp.	cornstarch
	Zest of one lemon
1/4 tsp.	tarragon
1/4 tsp.	salt
	Pepper to taste

- Heat chicken broth. Mix lemon juice and cornstarch together. Add the hot broth and zest. Let simmer on low heat until thickening, stirring. Season with tarragon, salt and pepper.
- Delicious on fish brochettes or poached fillets.

Mushroom sauce

4 TO 6 SERVINGS

(MICROWAVE OR TRADITIONAL METHOD)

NUTRITIONAL VALUE PER 1 TBSP. SERVING

	Amount	% DV
Calories	40	
Fat	2 g	3%
Saturated	0.5 g	2%
+ Trans	0 g	
Polyunsaturated	0.5 g	
Omega-6	0.3 g	
Omega-3 (ALA)	0.1 g	
Omega-3 (EPA+DHA)	0 g	
Monounsaturated	1 g	
Cholesterol	0 mg	0%
Sodium	95 mg	4%
Potassium	158 mg	5%
Carbohydrate	5 g	2%
Dietary Fibre	1 g	4%
Sugars	2 g	
Protein	1.5 g	
Vitamin A		1%
Vitamin C		6%
Calcium		1%
Iron		3%
Vitamin D		5%
Vitamin E		5%

DIABETIC EXCHANGE

None

2 tsp.	olive oil
1	finely chopped onion
1	crushed garlic clove
2 tsp.	cornstarch
3/4 cup (180 ml)	home-made beef broth (see recipe, p. 112) or fat-free salt-free commercial broth
2 tbsp.	tomato paste
1 pinch	*herbes de Provence* (see recipe, p. 259)
1/4 tsp.	salt
1 pinch	pepper
1 cup (250 ml)	fresh sliced mushrooms

Microwave method:

- In a 2 cup (500 ml) microwave-safe bowl, mix oil, onion and garlic. Cover and cook for 3 minutes at high intensity (10).
- Dissolve cornstarch in broth. Pour into the previous mixture. Add tomato paste and seasonings. Cook uncovered at high intensity for 2 minutes. Stir. Add mushrooms and cook uncovered for 3 minutes, stirring twice or until sauce is creamy.

Traditional method:

- In a frying pan, heat oil and margarine. Add onion and garlic. Cook on low for 5 minutes without letting it brown. Add broth and tomato paste. Bring to a boil. Add mushrooms and seasonings. Let simmer on low heat for 3 minutes. Add the cornstarch mixed with 2 tbsp. cold water. Cook until it thickens.

Note This simple, quickly-prepared sauce is exquisite on hamburgers, meatloaf, or tournedos from which the visible fat has been removed.

Mint sauce

4 SERVINGS

NUTRITIONAL VALUE PER 1 TBSP. SERVING		
	Amount	% DV
Calories	20	
Fat	0 g	0%
Saturated	0 g	0%
+ Trans	0 g	
Polyunsaturated	0 g	
Omega-6	0 g	
Omega-3 (ALA)	0 g	
Omega-3 (EPA+DHA)	0 g	
Monounsaturated	0 g	
Cholesterol	0 mg	0%
Sodium	2 mg	1%
Potassium	52 mg	2%
Carbohydrate	5 g	2%
Dietary Fibre	0 g	1%
Sugars	4 g	
Protein	0 g	
Vitamin A		1%
Vitamin C		26%
Calcium		1%
Iron		3%
Vitamin D		0%
Vitamin E		1%

DIABETIC EXCHANGE
None

1/2 cup (125 ml)	unsweetened apple juice
1 tsp.	red wine vinegar
1 tbsp.	lemon juice
1 tsp.	lemon zest
1 tbsp.	chopped fresh mint or 1 tsp. dried mint
1 tsp.	cornstarch

- Bring to a boil apple juice, vinegar, lemon juice, lemon zest, and mint. Simmer 2 minutes. Thicken with the cornstarch mixed with 1 tbsp. cold water.
- Serve on lamp chops or medallions.

Vegetable spaghetti sauce
MAKES 5 CUPS (1.25 LITRE)

NUTRITIONAL VALUE
PER ½ CUP (125 ML) SERVING

	Amount	% DV
Calories	65	
Fat	3 g	5%
Saturated	0.5 g	3%
+ Trans	0 g	
Polyunsaturated	1 g	
Omega-6	0.9 g	
Omega-3 (ALA)	0 g	
Omega-3 (EPA+DHA)	0 g	
Monounsaturated	1.5 g	
Cholesterol	0 mg	0%
Sodium	200 mg	9%
Potassium	274 mg	8%
Carbohydrate	9 g	4%
Dietary Fibre	1.5 g	7%
Sugars	4 g	
Protein	1 g	
Vitamin A		15%
Vitamin C		51%
Calcium		4%
Iron		7%
Vitamin D		0%
Vitamin E		10%

DIABETIC EXCHANGE

2 vegetables & fruits exchanges
½ oils & fats exchange

2 tbsp.	olive oil
2 cups (500 ml)	chopped leeks (both white and green parts)
1	large chopped onion
2	chopped garlic cloves
1 cup (250 ml)	grated broccoli stems
½ cup (125 ml)	chopped celery
1 ½ cup (275 ml)	grated carrots
2 ½ cups (625 ml)	tomato or vegetable juice
1 tsp.	fat-free salt-free instant soup base
1 tsp.	Worcestershire sauce
½ tsp.	pepper

- Heat oil in a heavy cooking pot. Sauté leeks with onion and garlic until they "perspire". Cook 4 to 5 minutes. Add vegetables, tomato juice and seasonings.
- Cook at medium-low heat for 1 hour, stirring often. Serve on spaghetti or fettuccine.

Note This sauce is equally delicious on sliced meatloaf and lean hamburger patties. It freezes very well.

Orange sauce
4 SERVINGS

NUTRITIONAL VALUE PER 5 TBSP. SERVING		
	Amount	% DV
Calories	30	
Fat	0.3 g	0%
Saturated	0.1 g	0%
+ Trans	0 g	
Polyunsaturated	0.1 g	
Omega-6	0 g	
Omega-3 (ALA)	0 g	
Omega-3 (EPA+DHA)	0 g	
Monounsaturated	0.1 g	
Cholesterol	0 mg	0%
Sodium	11 mg	1%
Potassium	95 mg	3%
Carbohydrate	6 g	2%
Dietary Fibre	0 g	1%
Sugars	3 g	
Protein	1 g	
Vitamin A		1%
Vitamin C		29%
Calcium		1%
Iron		2%
Vitamin D		0%
Vitamin E		1%

DIABETIC EXCHANGE
None

¹/₂ cup (125 ml)	home-made chicken broth (see recipe, p. 113) or fat-free salt-free commercial chicken broth
¹/₂ cup (125 ml)	fresh orange juice
¹/₄ cup (60 ml)	water
1 tbsp.	cornstarch
¹/₂ tsp.	orange zest
¹/₂ tsp.	fresh chopped marjoram
¹/₂ tsp.	fresh chopped thyme
2 tsp.	low-calorie sweetener (Splenda)

- Heat chicken broth and orange juice. Mix water with cornstarch and pour into the hot broth. Add zest.
- Cook over low heat until sauce thickens, stirring constantly. Season with marjoram and thyme. Add sweetener.

Instant tomato sauce
MAKES 2 ¹/₂ CUPS (625 ML)

NUTRITIONAL VALUE PER ¹/₂ CUP (125 ML) SERVING		
	Amount	% DV
Calories	35	
Fat	0.2 g	0%
Saturated	0 g	0%
+ Trans	0 g	
Polyunsaturated	0.1 g	
Omega-6	0.1 g	
Omega-3 (ALA)	0 g	
Omega-3 (EPA+DHA)	0 g	
Monounsaturated	0 g	
Cholesterol	0 mg	0%
Sodium	384 mg	16%
Potassium	283 mg	9%
Carbohydrate	7 g	3%
Dietary Fibre	1.5 g	7%
Sugars	5 g	
Protein	1 g	
Vitamin A		9%
Vitamin C		29%
Calcium		5%
Iron		10%
Vitamin D		0%
Vitamin E		9%

DIABETIC EXCHANGE

1 vegetables & fruits exchange

19 oz (540 ml)	diced canned tomatoes
2	chopped garlic cloves
1	small chopped onion
¹/₂ cup (125 ml)	sliced carrots
¹/₃ cup (80 ml)	sliced celery
¹/₂ tsp.	thyme
¹/₂ tsp.	salt
1 pinch	black pepper

- Put tomatoes and their juice through the mixer. Pour into a saucepan. Add garlic, onion, carrot and celery and cook at low heat until tender. Put through the mixer again. Season.

Fresh home-made tomato sauce

MAKES 6 CUPS (1.5 LITRE)

4 lb (2 kg)	coarsely chopped tomatoes
2	garlic cloves
1 cup (250 ml)	coarsely chopped green onions
1	sliced carrot
2	coarsely chopped celery stalks
¼ tsp.	tarragon
¼ tsp.	thyme
½ tsp.	savory
½ tsp.	salt
¼ tsp.	pepper

- Remove stems and put tomatoes through the food processor with the garlic, green onions, carrot and celery. Transfer everything into a large saucepan. Add tarragon, thyme and savory. Bring to a full boil. Reduce heat and simmer for about 2 hours or until the sauce has the desired consistency. Add salt and pepper.
- Put the sauce through the blender, about 2 cups (500 ml) at a time. Pour into small containers ½ to 1 cup maximum (125 to 250 ml) and store in the freezer. The frozen sauce thaws quickly in the microwave or on the stove at low heat.
- The recipe can be doubled if you wish.

Yogourt-cheese dip

MAKES 3/4 CUP (180 ML)

NUTRITIONAL VALUE PER 1 TBSP. SERVING		
	Amount	% DV
Calories	30	
Fat	0.5 g	1%
Saturated	0.1 g	0%
+ Trans	0 g	
Polyunsaturated	0.2 g	
Omega-6	0.2 g	
Omega-3 (ALA)	0 g	
Omega-3 (EPA+DHA)	0 g	
Monounsaturated	0.1 g	
Cholesterol	1 mg	1%
Sodium	99 mg	5%
Potassium	111 mg	4%
Carbohydrate	4 g	2%
Dietary Fibre	0 g	1%
Sugars	4 g	
Protein	2 g	
Vitamin A		1%
Vitamin C		2%
Calcium		7%
Iron		1%
Vitamin D		2%
Vitamin E		2%

DIABETIC EXCHANGE
None

- A recipe made from my home-made yogourt cheese (see recipe page 108), seasoned with chives or hot red pepper.
- This cheese makes an excellent dip if you add 1 tbsp. of light cholesterol-free salad dressing and 2 tbsp. chili sauce.
- Stir well to obtain a creamy consistency.
- Serve with raw vegetables: carrot sticks, celery strips, broccoli and cauliflower flowerets, mushroom caps.

215
Salads and salad dressings

Celeriac (celery root) salad

4 SERVINGS

NUTRITIONAL VALUE PER SERVING

	Amount	% DV
Calories	100	
Fat	4 g	6%
Saturated	0.5 g	3%
+ Trans	0 g	
Polyunsaturated	2.5 g	
Omega-6	2.2 g	
Omega-3 (ALA)	0.2 g	
Omega-3 (EPA+DHA)	0 g	
Monounsaturated	1 g	
Cholesterol	1 mg	0%
Sodium	465 mg	21%
Potassium	294 mg	8%
Carbohydrate	15 g	2%
Dietary Fibre	2 g	7%
Sugars	9 g	
Protein	2 g	
Vitamin A		13%
Vitamin C		13%
Calcium		5%
Iron		5%
Vitamin D		1%
Vitamin E		11%

DIABETIC EXCHANGE

1 1/2 vegetables & fruits exchange
1/2 meat & alternatives exchange

1/2	celeriac
1 tbsp.	lime juice
1	medium grated carrot
1	red apple, unpeeled and diced
2 tbsp.	raisins

DRESSING:

3 tbsp.	light mayonnaise
2 tbsp.	fat-free yogourt
1/2 tbsp.	Dijon mustard
1/2 tsp.	salt
1/2 tsp.	poppy seed
	Pepper to taste

- Peel the celeriac and grate finely. Add lime juice, mix well. Add grated carrot, diced apple and raisins.
- Combine dressing ingredients and mix into the grated celeriac. Refrigerate several hours before serving.

Marinated cucumber salad

8 SERVINGS

NUTRITIONAL VALUE PER SERVING

	Amount	% DV
Calories	80	
Fat	7 g	11%
Saturated	1 g	5%
+ Trans	0 g	
Polyunsaturated	1 g	
Omega-6	0.7 g	
Omega-3 (ALA)	0.1 g	
Omega-3 (EPA+DHA)	0 g	
Monounsaturated	5 g	
Cholesterol	0 mg	0%
Sodium	167 mg	7%
Potassium	141 mg	5%
Carbohydrate	5 g	2%
Dietary Fibre	1 g	4%
Sugars	3 g	
Protein	0.5 g	
Vitamin A		1%
Vitamin C		5%
Calcium		2%
Iron		3%
Vitamin D		0%
Vitamin E		11%

DIABETIC EXCHANGE

1 vegetables & fruits exchange
1/2 oils & fats exchange

2/3 cup (160 ml)	white wine vinegar
1/4 cup (60 ml)	olive oil
2 tbsp.	low-calorie sweetener (Splenda)
1 tsp.	basil
1 tsp.	Dijon mustard
1/2 tsp.	salt
8	peppercorns
1	finely chopped garlic clove
1	English cucumber
2	celery stalks
1	red onion

- In a salad bowl combine vinegar, oil, sweetener, basil, mustard, salt, peppercorns and garlic. Mix well.
- Slice unpeeled cucumber. Cut celery into diagonal slices and the onion into rings.
- Mix vegetables with the dressing. Cover and marinate for several hours. Remove peppercorns, drain and serve.

Couscous salad

4 SERVINGS

NUTRITIONAL VALUE PER SERVING		
	Amount	% DV
Calories	170	
Fat	4 g	6%
Saturated	0.5 g	3%
+ Trans	0 g	
Polyunsaturated	0.5 g	
Omega-6	0.4 g	
Omega-3 (ALA)	0.1 g	
Omega-3 (EPA+DHA)	0 g	
Monounsaturated	2.5 g	
Cholesterol	0 mg	0%
Sodium	141 mg	6%
Potassium	304 mg	9%
Carbohydrate	30 g	11%
Dietary Fibre	2 g	8%
Sugars	10 g	
Protein	4 g	
Vitamin A		4%
Vitamin C		61%
Calcium		4%
Iron		9%
Vitamin D		0%
Vitamin E		7%

DIABETIC EXCHANGE

1 vegetables & fruits exchange
1 1/2 grain product exchange
1/2 oils & fats exchange

3/4 cup (180 ml)	fresh orange juice
1/2 cup (125 ml)	couscous
1/4 cup (60 ml)	raisins
1/2 cup (125 ml)	finely chopped celery
2	chopped green onions
1/3 cup (80 ml)	chopped parsley
1 tbsp.	lemon juice
1 tbsp.	water
1 tbsp.	olive oil
1/4 tsp.	cumin
1/4 tsp.	curry
1/4 tsp.	salt
	Pepper to taste

- Bring orange juice to a boil. Add couscous. Cover and remove from heat. Let sit for 5 minutes.
- Stir and fluff the couscous with a fork. Add raisins, celery, onion and parsley.
- In a small bowl, whisk lemon juice, water, oil, cumin, curry, salt and pepper. Pour over couscous and mix well.

Note This salad can be served hot or cold.

Spinach grapefruit salad

4 SERVINGS

NUTRITIONAL VALUE PER SERVING

	Amount	% DV
Calories	170	
Fat	10.5 g	17%
Saturated	1.5 g	8%
+ Trans	0 g	
Polyunsaturated	1.2 g	
Omega-6	1 g	
Omega-3 (ALA)	0.2 g	
Omega-3 (EPA+DHA)	0 g	
Monounsaturated	7.5 g	
Cholesterol	0 mg	0%
Sodium	188 mg	8%
Potassium	674 mg	20%
Carbohydrate	16 g	6%
Dietary Fibre	3.5 g	15%
Sugars	2 g	
Protein	4 g	
Vitamin A		42%
Vitamin C		119%
Calcium		10%
Iron		19%
Vitamin D		0%
Vitamin E		33%

DIABETIC EXCHANGE

2 oils & fats exchanges
1 1/2 vegetables & fruits exchange

2	grapefruit
1	bag fresh spinach
1	red onion, sliced and separated into rings

DRESSING:

3 tbsp.	olive oil
1 tbsp.	raspberry vinegar
1	chopped garlic clove
1/4 tsp.	salt
	Pepper to taste

- Trim spinach. Put in a salad bowl.
- Remove skin and pith from the grapefruit. Cut the sections between the membranes and separate into four parts.
- Add to the spinach along with the onion rings.
- Mix dressing and add to salad. Mix well. Serve.

Gala salad

8 SERVINGS

NUTRITIONAL VALUE PER SERVING

	Amount	% DV
Calories	150	
Fat	11 g	17%
Saturated	1.5 g	8%
+ Trans	0 g	
Polyunsaturated	1.2 g	
Omega-6	1.1 g	
Omega-3 (ALA)	0.1 g	
Omega-3 (EPA+DHA)	0 g	
Monounsaturated	7.5 g	
Cholesterol	0 mg	0%
Sodium	281 mg	12%
Potassium	353 mg	11%
Carbohydrate	10 g	4%
Dietary Fibre	4.5 g	18%
Sugars	2 g	
Protein	3 g	
Vitamin A		1%
Vitamin C		19%
Calcium		4%
Iron		12%
Vitamin D		5%
Vitamin E		16%

DIABETIC EXCHANGE

2 oils & fats exchanges
2 vegetables & fruits exchanges

SALAD:

14 oz (398 ml)	canned hearts of palm
14 oz (398 ml)	canned artichoke hearts
1 cup (250 ml)	small whole mushrooms
1	avocado (optional)
1	red onion, sliced and separated into rings

DRESSING:

4	garlic cloves, crushed with a garlic press
1/4 cup (60 ml)	olive oil
2 tbsp.	raspberry vinegar
2 tbsp.	lemon juice or white wine
1/4 tsp.	salt
	Pepper to taste

- Rinse well and drain the hearts of palm and artichoke hearts. Clean small whole mushrooms thoroughly and add. Cut the hearts of palm and artichoke hearts into bite-sized pieces. Peel and slice avocado into small sections.
- Place all these ingredients in a salad bowl. Mix all dressing ingredients, sprinkle on the salad and gently toss.
- Chill well. Serve on lettuce leaves, decorated with red onion rings.
- This salad also makes a delicious starter, served on a lettuce leaf.

Note Marinated in their delicious dressing, the leftover vegetables will be just as tasty the next day.

Four seasons salad

6 SERVINGS

1 cup (250 ml)	spinach leaves
1	head of boston lettuce
1	small head of romaine
1/2	clove garlic

DRESSING:

1	finely chopped garlic clove
3 tbsp.	red wine vinegar
1/2 cup (125 ml)	walnut oil
2 tbsp.	dried tomatoes, chopped
1/4 tsp.	salt
	Pepper to taste
1/3 cup (80 ml)	walnut pieces

- Remove stems from spinach. Carefully wash spinach leaves and the two lettuces, then spin dry.
- Rub the sides of the salad bowl with the half-clove of garlic, place torn lettuce and spinach into the bowl by handfuls.
- In a small bowl, mix dressing ingredients. Refrigerate for several hours to allow the dried tomatoes to re-hydrate slightly. Just before serving, sprinkle dressing on the spinach and lettuce, and garnish with the walnut pieces.

Note Walnut oil is sold in supermarkets and health food stores. The taste is exquisite and it adds a very pleasant aroma to your salads.

NUTRITIONAL VALUE PER SERVING

	Amount	% DV
Calories	240	
Fat	23 g	35%
Saturated	2 g	12%
+ Trans	0 g	
Polyunsaturated	15.5 g	
Omega-6	12.8 g	
Omega-3 (ALA)	2.7 g	
Omega-3 (EPA+DHA)	0 g	
Monounsaturated	5 g	
Cholesterol	0 mg	0%
Sodium	95 mg	4%
Potassium	298 mg	9%
Carbohydrate	5 g	2%
Dietary Fibre	2 g	8%
Sugars	2 g	
Protein	3 g	
Vitamin A		21%
Vitamin C		26%
Calcium		4%
Iron		10%
Vitamin D		0%
Vitamin E		4%

DIABETIC EXCHANGE

1 vegetables & fruits exchange
4 1/2 oils & fats exchanges

Refreshing salad

4 SERVINGS

NUTRITIONAL VALUE PER SERVING, WITH DRESSING

	Teneur	% VQ
Calories	165	
Fat	10.5 g	17%
Saturated	1.5 g	8%
+ Trans	0 g	
Polyunsaturated	1.2 g	
Omega-6	1 g	
Omega-3 (ALA)	0.1 g	
Omega-3 (EPA+DHA)	0 g	
Monounsaturated	7.5 g	
Cholesterol	0 mg	0%
Sodium	133 mg	6%
Potassium	331 mg	10%
Carbohydrate	16 g	6%
Dietary Fibre	2.5 g	11%
Sugars	12 g	
Protein	2 g	
Vitamin A		11%
Vitamin C		40%
Calcium		5%
Iron		8%
Vitamin D		4%
Vitamin E		18%

ÉCHANGE POUR DIABÉTIQUES

2 oils & fats exchanges
1 vegetables & fruits exchange

DRESSING:

3 tbsp.	olive oil
1 tbsp.	strawberry or raspberry vinegar
1/2 tsp.	Dijon mustard
1/4 tsp.	salt
1 pinch	pepper
1 envelope	low-calorie sweetener (Splenda)
2	chopped garlic cloves

SALAD:

1	boston lettuce, torn into bite-sized pieces
1/2 cup (125 ml)	sliced fresh mushrooms
1	apple, cubed
1	orange cut in sections
1 bunch	red grapes
	Fresh parsley to garnish

- In a salad bowl mix oil, vinegar, mustard, salt, pepper, garlic and sweetener.
- Add salad ingredients. Mix and serve immediately.

Chicken supper-salad

4 SERVINGS

NUTRITIONAL VALUE PER SERVING

	Amount	% DV
Calories	390	
Fat	22 g	35%
Saturated	5.5 g	29%
+ Trans	0 g	
Polyunsaturated	4 g	
Omega-6	3.6 g	
Omega-3 (ALA)	0.3 g	
Omega-3 (EPA+DHA)	0 g	
Monounsaturated	11.5 g	
Cholesterol	82 mg	28%
Sodium	702 mg	30%
Potassium	770 mg	22%
Carbohydrate	18 g	6%
Dietary Fibre	5 g	21%
Sugars	5 g	
Protein	31 g	
Vitamin A		10%
Vitamin C		75%
Calcium		14%
Iron		13%
Vitamin D		5%
Vitamin E		35%

DIABETIC EXCHANGE

1 vegetables & fruits exchange
4 meat & alternatives exchanges
6 oils & fats exchanges

2 cups (500 ml)	cooked chicken breast, diced
1	dried shallot, sliced and separated into rings
2	finely sliced celery stalks
1	ripe avocado cut in cubes
1/2	red pepper cut in cubes
1/2 cup (125 ml)	crumbled feta
1/4 cup (60 ml)	coarsely chopped pecans
6	sliced black olives
	Creamy curry dressing (see recipe, p. 226)
	Boston lettuce leaves

- In a salad bowl, mix all ingredients except lettuce. Gently incorporate the Creamy curry dressing. Serve the salad in 4 plates garnished with a leaf of lettuce.

Tomato salad

6 SERVINGS

NUTRITIONAL VALUE PER SERVING, WITH DRESSING		
	Teneur	% VQ
Calories	110	
Fat	7 g	11%
Saturated	1 g	6%
+ Trans	0 g	
Polyunsaturated	1 g	
Omega-6	0.9 g	
Omega-3 (ALA)	0.1 g	
Omega-3 (EPA+DHA)	0 g	
Monounsaturated	5 g	
Cholesterol	0 mg	0%
Sodium	221 mg	10%
Potassium	407 mg	12%
Carbohydrate	11 g	4%
Dietary Fibre	2 g	9%
Sugars	1 g	
Protein	2 g	
Vitamin A		6%
Vitamin C		32%
Calcium		2%
Iron		9%
Vitamin D		0%
Vitamin E		16%

ÉCHANGE POUR DIABÉTIQUES

1 oils & fats exchange
1 vegetables & fruits exchange

5	good-sized red tomatoes
3	garlic cloves
2	green onions
1	dried shallot
½ tsp.	dried oregano or 1 tbsp. fresh basil
1 tsp.	dried parsley
½ tsp.	Dijon mustard
1 tbsp.	vinegar red wine
3 tbsp.	olive oil
½ tsp.	salt
	Pepper to taste

- Cut tomatoes in sections or thin slices. Chop garlic, green onion and shallot. Add to tomatoes with oregano and parsley.
- Mix mustard and vinegar, add oil, salt and pepper. Sprinkle on tomatoes.
- As a starter, serve on a lettuce leaf. This salad makes a nice addition to a cold buffet.

Garlic dressing

MAKES 3/4 CUP (180 ML)

NUTRITIONAL VALUE PER SERVING

	Amount	% DV
Calories	90	
Fat	9.5 g	15%
Saturated	1.5 g	7%
+ Trans	0 g	
Polyunsaturated	1 g	
Omega-6	0.9 g	
Omega-3 (ALA)	0.1 g	
Omega-3 (EPA+DHA)	0 g	
Monounsaturated	7 g	
Cholesterol	0 mg	0%
Sodium	46 mg	2%
Potassium	9 mg	1%
Carbohydrate	1 g	1%
Dietary Fibre	0 g	1%
Sugars	1 g	
Protein	0.5 g	
Vitamin A		1%
Vitamin C		3%
Calcium		1%
Iron		1%
Vitamin D		0%
Vitamin E		14%

DIABETIC EXCHANGE

2 oils & fats exchanges

1/2 cup (125 ml)	olive oil
2 tbsp.	lemon juice
4 tsp.	raspberry vinegar
1 tsp.	Dijon mustard
2	garlic cloves
1/2 tsp.	oregano
1/4 tsp.	salt
	Pepper to taste

- Mix all ingredients well. Keep in refrigerator in a tightly sealed jar. Shake well before serving.

Creamy curry dressing

MAKES 3/4 CUP (180 ML)

1/3 cup (80 ml)	light mayonnaise
1/3 cup (80 ml)	plain low-fat yogourt
1 tbsp.	lime juice
1 tsp.	fresh chopped basil
1 tsp.	curry
1/2 tsp.	salt
	Pepper to taste

- Mix all ingredients and keep dressing in the refrigerator in a tightly sealed container.

NUTRITIONAL VALUE PER 1 TBSP. SERVING

	Amount	% DV
Calories	30	
Fat	2.5 g	4%
Saturated	0.5 g	2%
+ Trans	0 g	
Polyunsaturated	1.5 g	
Omega-6	1.2 g	
Omega-3 (ALA)	0.1 g	
Omega-3 (EPA+DHA)	0 g	
Monounsaturated	0.5 g	
Cholesterol	3 mg	1%
Sodium	162 mg	7%
Potassium	23 mg	1%
Carbohydrate	2 g	1%
Dietary Fibre	0 g	1%
Sugars	1 g	
Protein	0 g	
Vitamin A		1%
Vitamin C		1%
Calcium		2%
Iron		1%
Vitamin D		1%
Vitamin E		3%
Vitamin K		3%

DIABETIC EXCHANGE

1/2 oils & fats exchange

Tarragon dressing

MAKES 1 1/2 CUPS (330 ML)

1 cup (250 ml)	olive oil
1/4 cup (60 ml)	tarragon vinegar
1/2 tsp.	dry mustard
1/2 tsp.	salt
1 envelope	low-calorie sweetener (Splenda)
1	crushed garlic clove
2 tbsp.	chopped chives
1 tsp.	chopped parsley
1/2 tsp.	tarragon

- Combine all ingredients in a jar with a tight-fitting lid. Shake well before serving.
- Store in refrigerator.

NUTRITIONAL VALUE PER 1 TBSP. SERVING

	Amount	% DV
Calories	95	
Fat	10 g	16%
Saturated	1.5 g	8%
+ Trans	0 g	
Polyunsaturated	1 g	
Omega-6	1 g	
Omega-3 (ALA)	0.1 g	
Omega-3 (EPA+DHA)	0 g	
Monounsaturated	7.5 g	
Cholesterol	0 mg	0%
Sodium	55 mg	3%
Potassium	7 mg	1%
Carbohydrate	0.5 g	1%
Dietary Fibre	0 g	1%
Sugars	1 g	
Protein	0 g	
Vitamin A		1%
Vitamin C		1%
Calcium		1%
Iron		1%
Vitamin D		0%
Vitamin E		15%

DIABETIC EXCHANGE

2 oils & fats exchanges

Italian-style dressing
MAKES 1 CUP (250 ML)

	Amount	% DV
NUTRITIONAL VALUE PER 1 TBSP. SERVING		
Calories	95	
Fat	10 g	16%
Saturated	1.5 g	8%
+ Trans	0 g	
Polyunsaturated	1 g	
Omega-6	1 g	
Omega-3 (ALA)	0.1 g	
Omega-3 (EPA+DHA)	0 g	
Monounsaturated	7.5 g	
Cholesterol	0 mg	0%
Sodium	35 mg	2%
Potassium	9 mg	1%
Carbohydrate	0.5 g	1%
Dietary Fibre	0 g	1%
Sugars	1 g	
Protein	0 g	
Vitamin A		1%
Vitamin C		1%
Calcium		1%
Iron		2%
Vitamin D		0%
Vitamin E		15%

DIABETIC EXCHANGE

2 oils & fats exchanges

1/4 cup (60 ml)	white wine vinegar
1 tsp.	Dijon mustard
3/4 cup (180 ml)	olive oil
2	minced garlic cloves
1 tsp.	chopped parsley
1 tsp.	oregano
1/4 tsp.	salt
1 pinch	pepper
1/8 tsp.	thyme
1/4 tsp.	paprika

- Whisk together vinegar, mustard and oil. Add remaining ingredients, mix well.
- Keep in refrigerator in a jar with a tight-fitting lid. Mix well before serving.
- This dressing is better if prepared 12 to 24 hours ahead of time.

Pink herb dressing
MAKE 1 1/4 CUP (330 ML)

NUTRITIONAL VALUE PER 1 TBSP. SERVING		
	Amount	% DV
Calories	25	
Fat	2.5 g	4%
Saturated	0.3 g	2%
+ Trans	0 g	
Polyunsaturated	0.3 g	
Omega-6	0.2 g	
Omega-3 (ALA)	0 g	
Omega-3 (EPA+DHA)	0 g	
Monounsaturated	2 g	
Cholesterol	0 mg	0%
Sodium	1 mg	1%
Potassium	16 mg	1%
Carbohydrate	1 g	1%
Dietary Fibre	0 g	1%
Sugars	1 g	
Protein	0 g	
Vitamin A		1%
Vitamin C		1%
Calcium		1%
Iron		1%
Vitamin D		0%
Vitamin E		4%

DIABETIC EXCHANGE
2 oils & fats exchanges

1 cup (250 ml)	strawberry, raspberry or red wine vinegar
1/4 cup (60 ml)	olive oil
3	garlic cloves, crushed, then finely chopped.
1 tbsp.	chopped chives
1 tsp.	fine herbs
3 envelopes	artificial sweetener (Splenda)

- Thoroughly mix all ingredients, mixing again just before serving.
- Delicious on green salad. Keep refrigerated.

231
Fruit

Mom's fruit candy

MAKES 24 CANDIES

¹/₂ cup (125 ml)	**dried pitted prunes**
¹/₂ cup (125 ml)	**pitted dates**
¹/₂ cup (125 ml)	**raisins**
1 tbsp.	**lemon juice**
¹/₄ cup (60 ml)	**unsweetened coconut, grated fine, or graham cracker crumbs**

- Put prunes, dates and raisins through a meat-grinder. Add lemon juice, mix well.
- Make little balls, about 1 inch (2.5 cm) in diameter, and roll in coconut or graham cracker crumbs. Keep in well- sealed container in refrigerator.

Note Here is a healthy little treat that contains neither fat nor added sugar.
It is rich in fibre, excellent for the intestines because fibre helps prevent constipation. But don't overdo it; too many of these candies can be too much of a good thing!

NUTRITIONAL VALUE PER SERVING (3 CANDIES)

	Amount	% DV
Calories	80	
Fat	2 g	4%
Saturated	1.7 g	9%
+ Trans 0 g		
Polyunsaturated	0 g	
Omega-6	0 g	
Omega-3 (ALA)	0 g	
Omega-3 (EPA+DHA)	0 g	
Monounsaturated	0.1 g	
Cholesterol	0 mg	0%
Sodium	3 mg	1%
Potassium	194 mg	6%
Carbohydrate	16.5 g	6%
Dietary Fibre	2 g	9%
Sugars	13 g	
Protein	1 g	
Vitamin A		1%
Vitamin C		3%
Calcium		2%
Iron		4%
Vitamin D		0%
Vitamin E		1%

DIABETIC EXCHANGE

1 vegetables & fruits exchange

Light strawberry jam

MAKES 3 - 1 CUP (250 ML) JARS

4 cups (1litre)	fresh or frozen strawberry pieces
2 tbsp.	lemon juice
1/2 cup (125 ml)	fresh orange juice
1 envelope	low-calorie strawberry gelatine powder (e.g. Jell-O Light)
1/3 cup (80 ml)	low-calorie sweetener (Splenda)
	A few drops of red food colouring

- Bring to a rolling boil: strawberries, lemon juice and orange juice. Remove from heat and add flavoured gelatine powder. Mix until it is completely dissolved.
- Bring to the boil again and cook for another minute.
- Remove from heat. Add sweetener and food colouring. Mix well.

Note This jam can be kept for 2 weeks in the refrigerator.

NUTRITIONAL VALUE PER 1 TBSP. SERVING

	Amount	% DV
Calories	5	
Fat	0 g	1%
Saturated	0 g	1%
+ Trans	0 g	
Polyunsaturated	0 g	
Omega-6	0 g	
Omega-3 (ALA)	0 g	
Omega-3 (EPA+DHA)	0 g	
Monounsaturated	0 g	
Cholesterol	0 mg	0%
Sodium	1 mg	1%
Potassium	26 mg	1%
Carbohydrate	1 g	1%
Dietary Fibre	0.5 g	2%
Sugars	1 g	
Protein	0 g	
Vitamin A		1%
Vitamin C		16%
Calcium		1%
Iron		1%
Vitamin D		0%
Vitamin E		1%

DIABETIC EXCHANGE

None

Raspberry coulis

MAKES 1 1/2 CUPS (300 ML)

10 oz (300 g)	unsweetened frozen raspberries
4 tsp.	low-calorie sweetener (Splenda)
1 tbsp.	Grand Marnier or Cointreau

- Purée raspberries in a blender or food processor. Strain through a sieve to remove seeds.
- Add sweetener, Grand Marnier or Cointreau. Refrigerate.

NUTRITIONAL VALUE PER 1 TBSP. SERVING

	Amount	% DV
Calories	10	
Fat	0 g	0%
Saturated	0 g	0%
+ Trans	0 g	
Polyunsaturated	0 g	
Omega-6	0 g	
Omega-3 (ALA)	0 g	
Omega-3 (EPA+DHA)	0 g	
Monounsaturated	0 g	
Cholesterol	0 mg	0%
Sodium	1 mg	1%
Potassium	23 mg	1%
Carbohydrate	2 g	1%
Dietary Fibre	1 g	4%
Sugars	2 g	
Protein	0 g	
Vitamin A		1%
Vitamin C		7%
Calcium		1%
Iron		1%
Vitamin D		0%
Vitamin E		2%

DIABETIC EXCHANGE

None

Sparkling strawberry juice

8 SERVINGS

NUTRITIONAL VALUE PER SERVING		
	Amount	% DV
Calories	50	
Fat	0 g	0%
Saturated	0 g	0%
+ Trans	0 g	
Polyunsaturated	0 g	
Omega-6	0 g	
Omega-3 (ALA)	0 g	
Omega-3 (EPA+DHA)	0 g	
Monounsaturated	0 g	
Cholesterol	0 mg	0%
Sodium	17 mg	1%
Potassium	217 mg	7%
Carbohydrate	12 g	5%
Dietary Fibre	1 g	5%
Sugars	9 g	
Protein	1 g	
Vitamin A		1%
Vitamin C		94%
Calcium		2%
Iron		5%
Vitamin D		0%
Vitamin E		2%

DIABETIC EXCHANGE
1 vegetables & fruits exchange

15 oz (450 g)	unsweetened frozen strawberries
3 drops	red food colouring
2 cups (500 ml)	fresh orange juice
3 cups (750 ml)	diet Seven-Up or Sprite

- Purée strawberries in the blender or food processor until liquid. Add food colouring, then the orange juice. Mix and allow to cool.
- Just before serving, add the diet soft drink. Serve in wine glasses with ice cubes containing a piece of orange zest.

Spring marmalade

MAKES 5 - 1 CUP (250 ML) JARS

6 cups (1.5 litre)	fresh rhubarb
19 oz (540 ml)	canned crushed unsweetened pineapple with juice
1 envelope	sugar-free strawberry gelatine powder (e.g. Jell-O Light)
1/2 cup (125 ml)	low-calorie sweetener (Splenda)

- Wash and chop rhubarb. In a large cooking pot, mix rhubarb with the canned pineapple and juice. Bring to a boil and cook 15 minutes, stirring occasionally.
- Remove from heat and add sugar-free strawberry gelatine powder and sweetener. Mix well. Cool and pour into jars. Allow to thoroughly cool, then freeze.

Note Like all sugar-free jams, this one has to be kept frozen. It freezes very well, so you can have some on hand all year round.

NUTRITIONAL VALUE PER 1 TBSP. SERVING

	Amount	% DV
Calories	5	
Fat	0 g	1%
Saturated	0 g	1%
+ Trans	0 g	
Polyunsaturated	0 g	
Omega-6	0 g	
Omega-3 (ALA)	0 g	
Omega-3 (EPA+DHA)	0 g	
Monounsaturated	0 g	
Cholesterol	0 mg	0%
Sodium	1 mg	1%
Potassium	35 mg	1%
Carbohydrate	1 g	1%
Dietary Fibre	0 g	1%
Sugars	1 g	
Protein	0 g	
Vitamin A		1%
Vitamin C		3%
Calcium		1%
Iron		1%
Vitamin D		0%
Vitamin E		1%

DIABETIC EXCHANGE

1/2 vegetables & fruits exchange

Baked apples

4 SERVINGS

(MICROWAVE OR TRADITIONAL METHOD)

NUTRITIONAL VALUE PER SERVING (1 APPLE)		
	Amount	% DV
Calories	125	
Fat	1 g	3%
Saturated	0 g	1%
+ Trans	0 g	
Polyunsaturated	1 g	
Omega-6	0.8 g	
Omega-3 (ALA)	0.2 g	
Omega-3 (EPA+DHA)	0 g	
Monounsaturated	0 g	
Cholesterol	0 mg	0%
Sodium	2 mg	1%
Potassium	271 mg	8%
Carbohydrate	29 g	10%
Dietary Fibre	3 g	13%
Sugars	23 g	
Protein	1 g	
Vitamin A		1%
Vitamin C		28%
Calcium		2%
Iron		4%
Vitamin D		0%
Vitamin E		2%

DIABETIC EXCHANGE

1 vegetables & fruits exchange
1/2 oils & fats exchange

2 tbsp.	raisins
3 tbsp.	chopped dates
1 tbsp.	chopped walnuts
4	cooking apples
	Juice of one orange (or two oranges, if following traditional method)

Microwave method:

- Mix raisins, dates and nuts.
- Core the apples and peel downwards until the halfway point.
- Place in a microwave-safe dish, peeled side up. Stuff each apple with the mixture of raisins, dates and nuts.
- Sprinkle with orange juice. Cook uncovered for 4 to 5 minutes at high intensity (10). Halfway through cooking, baste the apples with cooking juices. Let sit for 3 minutes after cooking. Serve hot or cold.

Traditional method:

- Heat oven to 375 °F (190 °C).
- Prepare apples in the same way as in the microwave recipe. Place in a shallow ovenproof dish, stuff with the mixture of raisins, dates and nuts, and sprinkle with the juice from the two oranges with water added, if necessary, to make 1/2 cup (125 ml) of liquid in all.
- Bake uncovered for 30 minutes. Baste the apples with sauce halfway through cooking time.

Note This recipe is a very good source of fibre.

Cranberry-orange relish

MAKES 2 - 1 CUP (250 ML) JARS

NUTRITIONAL VALUE PER 1 TBSP. SERVING

	Amount	% DV
Calories	15	
Fat	1 g	1%
Saturated	0 g	1%
+ Trans	0 g	
Polyunsaturated	0.5 g	
Omega-6	0.3 g	
Omega-3 (ALA)	0.1 g	
Omega-3 (EPA+DHA)	0 g	
Monounsaturated	0 g	
Cholesterol	0 mg	0%
Sodium	1 mg	1%
Potassium	32 mg	1%
Carbohydrate	3 g	1%
Dietary Fibre	0.5 g	3%
Sugars	1 g	
Protein	0 g	
Vitamin A		1%
Vitamin C		8%
Calcium		1%
Iron		1%
Vitamin D		0%
Vitamin E		1%

DIABETIC EXCHANGE

1/2 vegetables & fruits exchange

2 cups (500 ml)	fresh or frozen cranberries
1	orange, well washed
1/4 cup (60 ml)	chopped walnuts
1/3 cup (80 ml)	raisins
2/3 cup (160 ml)	low-calorie sweetener (Splenda)

- Put cranberries through a meat grinder while still frozen, that way they will not spatter. Next, grind the orange, complete with peel. Mix well. Add walnuts, raisins and sweetener. Stir. Cover and refrigerate for at least 24 hours before serving with turkey or chicken.

Note This relish keeps for 1 week in the refrigerator or several months in the freezer, in tightly-closed containers.

239

Desserts

Strawberry bars

9 SERVINGS

1	graham cracker pie-shell (see recipe, p. 244)
2 envelopes	flavourless gelatine
1/3 cup (80 ml)	cold water
2 cups (500 ml)	fresh chopped strawberries
1/2 cup (125 ml)	low-calorie sweetener (Splenda)
1 cup (250 ml)	plain fat-free yogourt
1 tbsp.	kirsch (optional)
1 tbsp.	lemon juice
2	egg whites
1/4 cup (60 ml)	chocolate chips
9	good-sized strawberries with stems, to garnish

- Prepare the graham cracker crumbs and press into a square 9-inch (22.5 cm) pan. Refrigerate.
- In a small bowl, let gelatine soak in cold water for 3 minutes.
- Meanwhile, reduce strawberries to a frothy purée in the food processor or blender.
- Melt gelatine in the microwave for 30 seconds at high intensity (10) or place bowl in a dish of boiling water. Stir until dissolved. Pour gelatine into the strawberry purée. Add sweetener, yogourt, kirsch and lemon juice. Cool until set.
- Beat egg whites to stiff peaks. Gently fold into strawberries. Pour the mixture onto the crust.
- Melt chocolate chips in the microwave oven at low intensity (3). Stir once a minute until they are completely melted. Dip the tip of each big strawberry into the chocolate and use them to decorate the strawberry cream.
- Refrigerate for a few hours or until strawberry cream is firm. Just before serving, cut into 9 squares.

Note The strawberry mixture can also be poured into a crown-shaped mould. Unmould just before serving and garnish with the chocolate-dipped strawberries.

NUTRITIONAL VALUE PER SERVING

	Amount	% DV
Calories	180	
Fat	9 g	15%
Saturated	1.5 g	9%
+ Trans	0.1 g	
Polyunsaturated	2.5 g	
Omega-6	1.8 g	
Omega-3 (ALA)	0.7 g	
Omega-3 (EPA+DHA)	0 g	
Monounsaturated	4.5 g	
Cholesterol	2 mg	1%
Sodium	112 mg	5%
Potassium	203 mg	4%
Carbohydrate	20 g	7%
Dietary Fibre	2 g	8%
Sugars	12 g	
Protein	5 g	
Vitamin A		1%
Vitamin C		58%
Calcium		7%
Iron		6%
Vitamin D		2%
Vitamin E		13%

DIABETIC EXCHANGE

1/2 vegetables & fruits exchange
1/2 grain product exchange
1 oils & fats exchange

Fruit Charlotte

8 SERVINGS

NUTRITIONAL VALUE PER SERVING		
	Amount	% DV
Calories	30	
Fat	0 g	1%
Saturated	0 g	1%
+ Trans	0 g	
Polyunsaturated	0 g	
Omega-6	0 g	
Omega-3 (ALA)	0 g	
Omega-3 (EPA+DHA)	0 g	
Monounsaturated	0 g	
Cholesterol	0 mg	0%
Sodium	75 mg	4%
Potassium	104 mg	3%
Carbohydrate	6 g	3%
Dietary Fibre	0 g	1%
Sugars	5 g	
Protein	2 g	
Vitamin A		1%
Vitamin C		37%
Calcium		1%
Iron		1%
Vitamin D		0%
Vitamin E		1%

DIABETIC EXCHANGE

1/2 vegetables & fruits exchange

1	envelope of flavourless gelatine
1/4 cup (60 ml)	cold water
1/2 cup (125 ml)	sugar-free pineapple juice
1/2 cup (125 ml)	low-calorie sweetener (Splenda)
1/4 tsp.	salt
2 tbsp.	lemon juice
1 cup (250 ml)	fresh orange juice
2	egg whites, beaten until they form stiff peaks

- Place the bowl and beaters of the electric mixer in the freezer so that they are thoroughly chilled, or quickly chill them by plunging them in cold water with ice cubes for 10 minutes. Drain. Soften the gelatine in cold water. Heat pineapple juice and dissolve gelatine in it. Add sweetener and salt, lemon and orange juice. Chill until partially set.
- Beat egg whites into stiff peaks.
- With the mixer, beat the fruit gelatine preparation until it is light and frothy. With a spatula, gently fold in beaten egg.
- Pour into a Charlotte mould or pan and garnish with pieces of pineapple, maraschino cherries and small fresh mint leaves.

Crème pâtissière (French pastry cream)

MAKES 2 CUPS (500 ML)
(MICROWAVE OR TRADITIONAL METHOD)

NUTRITIONAL VALUE PER ½ CUP (125 ML) SERVING		
	Amount	% DV
Calories	105	
Fat	3 g	5%
Saturated	1.5 g	7%
+ Trans	0.1 g	
Polyunsaturated	0 g	
Omega-6	0.2 g	
Omega-3 (ALA)	0 g	
Omega-3 (EPA+DHA)	0 g	
Monounsaturated	1 g	
Cholesterol	52 mg	18%
Sodium	210 mg	9%
Potassium	252 mg	8%
Carbohydrate	13 g	5%
Dietary Fibre	0 g	1%
Sugars	0 g	
Protein	7 g	
Vitamin A		10%
Vitamin C		3%
Calcium		18%
Iron		2%
Vitamin D		30%
Vitamin E		3%

DIABETIC EXCHANGE
½ milk & alternatives exchange

2 cups (500 ml)	1% milk
1	lightly beaten egg
3 tbsp.	cornstarch
¼ tsp.	salt
½ cup (125 ml)	low-calorie sweetener (Splenda)
1 tsp.	vanilla

Microwave method:

- In a 4-cup (1-litre) pyrex dish, heat the milk for 4 minutes at medium intensity (7).
- Combine egg, cornstarch and salt. Slowly add to hot milk. Cook 5 to 6 minutes at medium intensity (7), stirring 2 to 3 times, until it attains a thick creamy consistency.
- Remove from oven, stir, add sweetener and vanilla.
- Stretch a sheet of plastic wrap over the surface of the pastry cream to prevent a skin from forming. Let cool completely.

Traditional method:

- In a saucepan, mix cornstarch and salt. Add milk gradually. Cook over medium heat, stirring, until mixture has thickened.
- Pour a bit of milk into the beaten egg, whisking, then pour the egg into the hot milk mixture. Cook for another minute, beating with the whisk.
- Remove from heat, add vanilla and sweetener. Cool.

Orchard crepes

6 SERVINGS

NUTRITIONAL VALUE PER SERVING

	Amount	% DV
Calories	205	
Fat	4 g	7%
Saturated	1 g	6%
+ Trans	0.1 g	
Polyunsaturated	1 g	
Omega-6	0.8 g	
Omega-3 (ALA)	0.2 g	
Omega-3 (EPA+DHA)	0 g	
Monounsaturated	2 g	
Cholesterol	35 mg	12%
Sodium	156 mg	7%
Potassium	344 mg	10%
Carbohydrate	35 g	12%
Dietary Fibre	3.5 g	14%
Sugars	12 g	
Protein	8 g	
Vitamin A		6%
Vitamin C		10%
Calcium		14%
Iron		10%
Vitamin D		16%
Vitamin E		9%

DIABETIC EXCHANGE

1 vegetables & fruits exchange
1 grain product exchange
1/2 oils & fats exchange

CREPES:

1 recipe	Crepe mix (see recipe, p. 249)
1 tsp.	vanilla

FILLING:

4	apples, Spartan or Cortland
1 tbsp.	canola olive oil
1 tbsp.	low-calorie sweetener (Splenda)
1/2 tsp.	cinnamon
	Light vanilla yogourt or iced milk to garnish

- Prepare crepe mix, flavouring with the vanilla. Cook the crepes and keep warm in oven heated to 150 °F (70 °C). Makes 6 crepes.
- Prepare crepe filling. Peel and core apples and cut in thin slices.
- Heat the oil in a large non-stick frying pan. Sauté apples until tender, at medium heat, for 8 minutes. Add sweetener and cinnamon. Mix well.
- Spread apple mixture on each crepe and roll up into "cigars". Serve with light vanilla yogourt or a dab of ice-milk on top.

Graham cracker crumb pie-shell

MAKES 1 PIE SHELL

(MICROWAVE OR TRADITIONAL METHOD)

¹/₄ cup (60 ml)	canola oil
1 ¹/₄ cups (300 ml)	graham cracker crumbs

- Combine graham cracker crumbs with the oil. Press the mixture into a 9-inch (22.5 cm) pyrex pie pan, covering the bottom and sides.
- Bake at 375 °F (190 °C) for 8 minutes, or in the microwave at medium intensity (7) for 3 minutes.

NUTRITIONAL VALUE PER SERVING (¹/₆ OF CRUST)

	Amount	% DV
Calories	120	
Fat	8 g	13%
Saturated	0.5 g	5%
+ Trans	0.2 g	
Polyunsaturated	2.5 g	
Omega-6	1.9 g	
Omega-3 (ALA)	0.7 g	
Omega-3 (EPA+DHA)	0 g	
Monounsaturated	4.5 g	
Cholesterol	0 mg	0%
Sodium	81 mg	4%
Potassium	18 mg	3%
Carbohydrate	10 g	4%
Dietary Fibre	0.5 g	2%
Sugars	4 g	
Protein	1 g	
Vitamin A		0%
Vitamin C		0%
Calcium		1%
Iron		4%
Vitamin D		0%
Vitamin E		13%

DIABETIC EXCHANGE

1 grain product exchange
2 oils & fats exchanges

Summer almond fruit treat

6 SERVINGS

1 recipe	*Crème pâtissière* (French pastry cream) (see recipe, p. 242)
1 tsp.	almond essence
2 cups (500 ml)	fresh-sliced strawberries, raspberries or peaches
1/4 cup (60 ml)	low-calorie sweetener (Splenda)
1/4 cup (60 ml)	grilled flaked almonds

- Prepare pastry cream. Flavour with almond essence. Place a sheet of plastic wrap directly on the surface of the cream to prevent a skin from forming. Cool.
- Prepare the fruit. Add sweetener and mix well.
- Transfer fruit to six little dessert bowls and cover with pastry cream.
- Garnish with grilled flaked almonds and a big strawberry, whole or cut in a fan shape.

Berry delight

8 SERVINGS

	Amount	% DV
NUTRITIONAL VALUE PER SERVING		
Calories	45	
Fat	0 g	1%
Saturated	0 g	1%
+ Trans	0 g	
Polyunsaturated	0 g	
Omega-6	0.1 g	
Omega-3 (ALA)	0 g	
Omega-3 (EPA+DHA)	0 g	
Monounsaturated	0 g	
Cholesterol	1 mg	1%
Sodium	40 mg	2%
Potassium	155 mg	5%
Carbohydrate	8 g	3%
Dietary Fibre	1.5 g	7%
Sugars	5 g	
Protein	4 g	
Vitamin A		1%
Vitamin C		31%
Calcium		6%
Iron		2%
Vitamin D		2%
Vitamin E		3%

DIABETIC EXCHANGE

1/2 vegetables & fruits exchange

1 cup (250 ml)	fresh or frozen unsweetened strawberries
1 cup (250 ml)	fresh or frozen unsweetened raspberries
1/2 cup (125 ml)	fresh or frozen unsweetened blueberries
2 tbsp.	lemon juice
2 envelopes	flavourless gelatine
1/2 cup (125 ml)	cold water
1 cup (250 ml)	plain fat-free yogourt
2	egg whites
1/2 cup (125 ml)	low-calorie sweetener (Splenda)

- After defrosting the berries, reduce to a frothy purée in the blender or food processor. Add lemon juice. Set aside.
- In a small bowl, soak gelatine in cold water for 5 minutes. Melt in microwave for 30 seconds at high intensity (10) or set bowl in a dish filled with boiling water. Stir until it dissolves. Pour gelatine into the fruit purée. Mix well.
- Add yogourt, combine. Refrigerate until the mixture is partially set. Beat the egg whites until frothy.
- Add sweetener and continue beating egg whites until firm. Gently fold into the fruit mixture with a spatula.
- Apply non-stick vegetable spray to an attractive 5-cup (1.5-litre) mould. Pour mixture in the mould and refrigerate overnight. Unmould onto a serving plate, garnish with fresh strawberries or raspberries.

Mango lime mousse

8 SERVINGS

2 envelopes	flavourless gelatine
1/2 cup (125 ml)	cold water
3	ripe mangoes, peeled and pitted
1/2 cup (125 ml)	lime juice
	Zest of one lime
2	egg whites
1/2 cup (125 ml)	low-calorie sweetener (Splenda)
1 cup (250 ml)	plain fat-free yogourt
2 or 3 drops	green food colouring

- First, prepare a 4-cup (1-litre) soufflé dish by making a paper "collar" that will extend the rim of the dish upwards 3 inches (8 cm). Make the paper collar by folding a strip of wax paper in half lengthwise (the strip should be 6 inches /16 cm wide), spraying it on one side with non-stick vegetable spray. Using tape, attach it (sprayed side in) around the edge of the soufflé mould.
- In a small bowl, soak the gelatine in cold water for 5 minutes. Melt in microwave oven for 30 seconds at high intensity (10) or place the bowl in a dish of boiling water.
- Purée the mango pulp in the blender. Pour into a big bowl. Add melted gelatine, lime juice and zest. Refrigerate for about 30 minutes or until mixture has thickened slightly.
- Beat egg whites until frothy. Add sweetener and continue beating until stiff peaks are formed.
- Pour yogourt into the mango mixture, then gently fold in egg whites. Add colouring.
- Pour into the soufflé dish. Refrigerate overnight. Remove paper collar. Decorate as desired. Serve.

Note The mango and lime mousse mixture can also be poured into a Bavarois mould. Refrigerate overnight and unmould before serving. Garnish with thin slices of lime.

French toast

4 SERVINGS

NUTRITIONAL VALUE PER SERVING (1 SLICE)		
	Amount	% DV
Calories	125	
Fat	6 g	9%
Saturated	1.5 g	7%
+ Trans	0 g	
Polyunsaturated	1.2 g	
Omega-6	0.9 g	
Omega-3 (ALA)	0.3 g	
Omega-3 (EPA+DHA)	0 g	
Monounsaturated	3 g	
Cholesterol	48 mg	16%
Sodium	202 mg	9%
Potassium	126 mg	4%
Carbohydrate	14 g	5%
Dietary Fibre	2 g	8%
Sugars	6 g	
Protein	5 g	
Vitamin A		7%
Vitamin C		1%
Calcium		6%
Iron		8%
Vitamin D		17%
Vitamin E		4%

DIABETIC EXCHANGE

1 grain product exchange

1	egg
1/3 cup (80 ml)	1% milk
1/2 tsp.	vanilla
1/4 tsp.	nutmeg
	Margarine
4 slices	whole-wheat bread

- Beat egg with milk, vanilla and nutmeg.
- Spread a thin layer of margarine on one side of each slice of bread. Put them margarine side down in a large non-stick frying pan at medium heat.
- Pour a quarter of the egg mixture over each slice of bread, thoroughly coating. Flip slices over and cook on the other side.

Note Delicious served with Yogourt cheese (see recipe, p. 108) or with Light strawberry jam (see recipe, p. 233).

Crepe mix

6 SERVINGS

1	whole egg
1	egg white
1 1/2	cups (375 ml) 1% milk
1 cup (250 ml)	flour.
1/4 tsp.	salt

- Beat whole egg and egg white in a bowl. Add milk, mix in flour and salt.
- Spray a 10-inch (25 cm) non-stick frying pan with non-stick vegetable spray.
- Pour in 1/3 cup (80 ml) of crepe mix. Spread it over the bottom of the pan and cook on both sides at medium heat or until golden.

NUTRITIONAL VALUE PER SERVING

	Amount	% DV
Calories	125	
Fat	2 g	3%
Saturated	1 g	5%
+ Trans	0 g	
Polyunsaturated	0.3 g	
Omega-6	0.2 g	
Omega-3 (ALA)	0 g	
Omega-3 (EPA+DHA)	0 g	
Monounsaturated	0.5 g	
Cholesterol	34 mg	12%
Sodium	137 mg	6%
Potassium	190 mg	6%
Carbohydrate	20 g	7%
Dietary Fibre	1.5 g	7%
Sugars	1 g	
Protein	7 g	
Vitamin A		6%
Vitamin C		2%
Calcium		10%
Iron		8%
Vitamin D		16%
Vitamin E		3%

DIABETIC EXCHANGE

1/2 milk & alternatives exchange
1 grain product exchange

Fruity watermelon bowl

12 SERVINGS

NUTRITIONAL VALUE PER SERVING

	Amount	% DV
Calories	75	
Fat	0 g	1%
Saturated	0 g	1%
+ Trans	0 g	
Polyunsaturated	0 g	
Omega-6	0.1 g	
Omega-3 (ALA)	0 g	
Omega-3 (EPA+DHA)	0 g	
Monounsaturated 0 g		
Cholesterol	0 mg	0%
Sodium	22 mg	1%
Potassium	416 mg	12%
Carbohydrate	19 g	7%
Dietary Fibre	1.5 g	6%
Sugars	16 g	
Protein	2 g	
Vitamin A		10%
Vitamin C		70%
Calcium		2%
Iron		4%
Vitamin D		0%
Vitamin E		1%

DIABETIC EXCHANGE

1 vegetables & fruits exchange

1 of each	small watermelon, cantaloupe, honeydew melon
	Fresh fruit: strawberries, pears, peaches, kiwis, according to personal preference.
¹/₂ cup (125 ml)	fresh orange juice
2 envelopes	low-calorie sweetener (Splenda)
1 tbsp.	Grand Marnier or cognac (optional)

- Cut a wide opening in the watermelon and scoop out inside to make a bowl.
- Remove the inside of the watermelon with a melon scoop, making little balls, and repeat the process with the canteloupe and honeydew melons.
- Mix with the other fresh fruit and transfer into the watermelon shell.
- Mix fresh-squeezed orange juice, sweetener and Grand Marnier or cognac.
- Pour over the fruit. Keep cold until just before serving.

Rice and raisin pudding

6 SERVINGS

1 recipe	*Crème pâtissière* (see recipe, p. 242)
⅓ cup (80 ml)	raisins
1 ½ cups (375 ml)	cooked long-grain rice
1 pinch	nutmeg

- Prepare crème patissière. Cover raisins with boiling water for 2 minutes until they swell. Drain.
- Add rice to crème patissière along with the raisins.
- Pour into a serving dish and sprinkle with a pinch of nutmeg.

NUTRITIONAL VALUE PER SERVING

	Amount	% DV
Calories	150	
Fat	2 g	4%
Saturated	1 g	5%
+ Trans	0 g	
Polyunsaturated	0 g	
Omega-6	0.2 g	
Omega-3 (ALA)	0 g	
Omega-3 (EPA+DHA)	0 g	
Monounsaturated	0.5 g	
Cholesterol	35 mg	2%
Sodium	141 mg	6%
Potassium	255 mg	8%
Carbohydrate	27 g	9%
Dietary Fibre	1 g	4%
Sugars	6 g	
Protein	6 g	
Vitamin A		7%
Vitamin C		3%
Calcium		13%
Iron		4%
Vitamin D		20%
Vitamin E		2%

DIABETIC EXCHANGE

1 grain product exchange
½ milk & alternatives exchange

Mini fruit mousse with raspberry coulis

4 SERVINGS

1 envelope	flavourless gelatine
1/4 cup (60 ml)	cold water
1 1/2 cups (375 ml)	home-made or canned sugar-free apple sauce
1/4 cup (60 ml)	low-calorie sweetener (Splenda)
1 tbsp.	orange zest
2	oranges, skin and pith peeled off, cut into sections
	Raspberry coulis (see recipe, p. 234)

- Soak gelatine in cold water for 5 minutes. At low heat, stirring, heat apple sauce until it boils. Remove from heat. Add gelatine, stir until it melts. Let cool.
- Add sweetener, zest and orange sections. Pour into 4 individual moulds treated with non-stick vegetable spray. Refrigerate until they are set. Unmould.
- Drizzle a bit of rasberry coulis over each serving plate and place apple mousse on top.

NUTRITIONAL VALUE PER SERVING

	Amount	% DV
Calories	135	
Fat	1 g	1%
Saturated	0 g	1%
+ Trans	0 g	
Polyunsaturated	0.5 g	
Omega-6	0.2 g	
Omega-3 (ALA)	0.1 g	
Omega-3 (EPA+DHA)	0 g	
Monounsaturated	0 g	
Cholesterol	0 mg	0%
Sodium	7 mg	1%
Potassium	308 mg	9%
Carbohydrate	30 g	10%
Dietary Fibre	7.5 g	30%
Sugars	21 g	
Protein	3 g	
Vitamin A		1%
Vitamin C		111%
Calcium		5%
Iron		6%
Vitamin D		0%
Vitamin E		10%

DIABETIC EXCHANGE

2 vegetables & fruits exchanges

Cold raspberry soufflé

8 SERVINGS

NUTRITIONAL VALUE PER SERVING

	Amount	% DV
Calories	70	
Fat	1 g	2%
Saturated	0.5 g	2%
+ Trans	0 g	
Polyunsaturated	0 g	
Omega-6	0.2 g	
Omega-3 (ALA)	0.1 g	
Omega-3 (EPA+DHA)	0 g	
Monounsaturated	0 g	
Cholesterol	2 mg	1%
Sodium	53 mg	3%
Potassium	205 mg	6%
Carbohydrate	11 g	4%
Dietary Fibre	3.5 g	15%
Sugars	6 g	
Protein	6 g	
Vitamin A		1%
Vitamin C		34%
Calcium		8%
Iron		4%
Vitamin D		0%
Vitamin E		6%

DIABETIC EXCHANGE

1 vegetables & fruits exchange

2 envelopes	flavourless gelatine
1/3 cup (80 ml)	fresh orange juice
3 cups (750 ml)	unsweetened frozen raspberries or 3 1/2 cups (875 ml) fresh raspberries
1 tsp.	grated orange zest
4	egg whites
1 cup (250 ml)	home-made yogourt or commercial low-fat yogourt
2/3 cup (160 ml)	low-calorie sweetener (Splenda)

- Prepare a 4-cup (1-litre) soufflé dish by taping a paper collar onto it. It must raise the edge of the dish by 3 inches (8 cm). Make the collar from a double layer of wax paper sprayed with non-stick vegetable spray.
- Soak gelatine in the orange juice for 3 minutes. Melt in the microwave, 30 seconds at high intensity (10), or by putting the dish in a saucepan with a few inches of boiling water.
- Defrost raspberries if necessary and purée in a food processor or blender.
- Transfer to a large bowl. Add dissolved gelatine and orange zest. Cool for about 30 minutes or until it thickens slightly.
- Beat egg whites in a large bowl until they are frothy. Add sweetener and continue beating until they form stiff peaks. Mix yogourt into the raspberry preparation. Using a spatula, gently fold in egg whites.
- Pour into the soufflé dish. Refrigerate at least 6 hours. Remove paper collar. Garnish with fresh raspberries and thin slices of orange.

Banana cream pie

6 SERVINGS

NUTRITIONAL VALUE PER SERVING (¹/₆ PIE)

	Amount	% DV
Calories	290	
Fat	15 g	24%
Saturated	2 g	12%
+ Trans	0.3 g	
Polyunsaturated	4.5 g	
Omega-6	3.2 g	
Omega-3 (ALA)	1.2 g	
Omega-3 (EPA+DHA)	0 g	
Monounsaturated	8.5 g	
Cholesterol	35 mg	12%
Sodium	257 mg	11%
Potassium	342 mg	10%
Carbohydrate	32 g	11%
Dietary Fibre	1 g	5%
Sugars	11 g	
Protein	6 g	
Vitamin A		7%
Vitamin C		12%
Calcium		13%
Iron		7%
Vitamin D		20%
Vitamin E		23%

DIABETIC EXCHANGE

1 vegetables & fruits exchange
1 grain product exchange
¹/₂ milk & alternatives exchange

1	graham cracker crumb pie-shell (see recipe, p. 244)

FILLING:

3 tbsp.	cornstarch
¹/₄ tsp.	salt
2 cups (500 ml)	1% milk
1	lightly beaten egg white
1	whole egg, beaten
1 tbsp.	margarine
1 tsp.	almond essence
¹/₂ cup (125 ml)	low-calorie sweetener (Splenda)

GARNISH:

2	sliced bananas
2 tbsp.	lemon juice

- Prepare pie-shell. Chill.
- Filling: In a non-stick saucepan, mix cornstarch and salt. Gradually whisk in the milk. Keep stirring over medium heat until the mixture boils. Continue cooking for another 2 minutes.
- Remove from heat. Dribble a bit of the hot mixture into the beaten eggs. Continue stirring and pour eggs into the hot milk mixture. Cook for another 2 minutes while stirring. Remove from heat, add margarine, almond essence and sweetener.
- Place a sheet of plastic wrap directly on the surface of the cream to prevent a skin from forming. Allow to thoroughly cool.
- Pour half of the cooled cream into the pie shell. Slice 1 ¹/₂ bananas and arrange slices on top, then cover with remaining cream.
- Garnish with slices of the remaining half-banana soaked in lemon juice.

Fruit cream pie

6 SERVINGS

NUTRITIONAL VALUE PER SERVING (¹/6 PIE)

	Amount	% DV
Calories	275	
Fat	13 g	21%
Saturated	2 g	11%
+ Trans	0.3 g	
Polyunsaturated	3.5 g	
Omega-6	2.8 g	
Omega-3 (ALA)	1 g	
Omega-3 (EPA+DHA)	0 g	
Monounsaturated	7 g	
Cholesterol	35 mg	12%
Sodium	249 mg	11%
Potassium	322 mg	10%
Carbohydrate	33 g	12%
Dietary Fibre	2.5 g	11%
Sugars	13 g	
Protein	6 g	
Vitamin A		7%
Vitamin C		46%
Calcium		14%
Iron		8%
Vitamin D		20%
Vitamin E		24%

DIABETIC EXCHANGE

2 oils & fats exchanges
1 grain product exchange
1 vegetables & fruits exchange
¹/2 milk & alternatives exchange

1	graham cracker crumb pie-shell (see recipe, p. 244)
1 recipe	*Crème pâtissière* (French pastry cream) (see recipe p. 242)
	Fresh fruit: kiwis, grapes, blueberries, peaches, pears, etc., according to preference

GLAZE:

¹/3 cup (80 ml)	water
2 tsp.	arrowroot or cornstarch
2 envelopes	artificial sweetener
1 tsp.	lemon juice
1 tsp.	sugar-free lemon-flavoured gelatine powder (for colour)

- Prepare graham cracker pie-shell and *crème pâtissière*.
- When the crème has cooled, pour into the pie-shell. Decorate with the fruit.
- Prepare the glaze. Mix together water and arrowroot in a measuring cup. Stir, then cook at high intensity (10) for 40 seconds in the microwave. Stir again and cook for another 30 seconds or until it thickens. Add sweetener, lemon juice and sugar-free gelatine. Combine well.
- Pour or brush over the fruit with a pastry brush. Refrigerate.

Fresh strawberry pie

6 SERVINGS

3 cups (750 ml)	fresh strawberries
1	graham cracker crumb pie-shell (see recipe, p. 244)
1 envelope	sugar-free strawberry gelatine powder
2 cups (500 ml)	boiling water
2 tbsp.	arrowroot or cornstarch

- Arrange the fresh strawberries over the bottom of the pie-shell.
- Bring to a boil the sugar-free gelatine powder, water and arrowroot. Cook until it becomes translucent.
- Cool and pour into the pie crust.
- Allow to completely cool.

NUTRITIONAL VALUE PER SERVING (¹/₆ PIE)

	Amount	% DV
Calories	200	
Fat	11 g	18%
Saturated	1 g	6%
+ Trans	0.2 g	
Polyunsaturated	3.5 g	
Omega-6	2.6 g	
Omega-3 (ALA)	1 g	
Omega-3 (EPA+DHA)	0 g	
Monounsaturated	6.5 g	
Cholesterol	0 mg	0%
Sodium	111 mg	5%
Potassium	148 mg	5%
Carbohydrate	22 g	8%
Dietary Fibre	2.5 g	10%
Sugars	9 g	
Protein	3 g	
Vitamin A		1%
Vitamin C		79%
Calcium		2%
Iron		8%
Vitamin D		0%
Vitamin E		20%

DIABETIC EXCHANGE

2 oils & fats exchanges
1 grain product exchange
1 vegetables & fruits exchange
¹/₂ milk & alternatives exchange

257

A few tasty tips

Healthy seasoning (Salt substitute)

MAKES 6 TBSP. (90 ML)

5 tsp.	onion powder
1 tbsp.	paprika
1 tbsp.	garlic powder
1 tbsp.	mustard powder
1 tsp.	basil
1 tsp.	marjoram
1 tsp.	rosemary
½ tsp.	pepper
¼ tsp.	savory
¼ tsp.	celery seeds

- In a small bowl, mix ingredients (take extra care with crushing the celery seeds). Pour into a salt shaker.

Herbes de Provence
MAKES $^1/2$ CUP (125 ML)

3 tbsp.	thyme
8	crushed bay leaves
2 tbsp.	ground rosemary
2 tbsp.	basil
1 tbsp.	savory
1 tsp.	ground fennel seeds

- Mix all ingredients together, grinding them evenly in a food processor.
- Keep in a well-marked spice jar.
- *Herbes de Provence* give an exquisite flavor to grilled and braised meat. They also make a perfect seasoning for vegetables, soups and fish.
- They can be hard to find, except at specialty grocery stores or import counters. But they are easy to prepare yourself, and they are fantastic!

Note If you don't have a food processor, ingredients can be put in a little plastic bag and crushed with a rolling pin. But naturally the herbs will not be as evenly ground.

Strawberry or raspberry vinegar

Makes 2 cups (500 ml)

1 cup (250 ml)	fruit, strawberries or raspberries
1 cup (250 ml)	white wine vinegar

- Trim and wash berries, putting them in a 2-cup (500 ml) Mason-type jar. Add vinegar. Allow to steep for 1 month in a darkened room.
- Filter the vinegar with a piece of cotton. Pour into a bottle with a tight-fitting top.
- Keep stored in a dry cool place.
- This is a delicious vinegar, and easy to make at home. Take advantage of summer to stock up on fresh berries. If necessary, fresh berries can be replaced by frozen ones (defrosted and drained). But the result is a little different.

Recipe index

Bibliography

MC PHERSON R., J. FROLICH, G. FODOR, J. GENEST, "Recommendations for the diagnostic and treatment of dyslipidemias and cardiovascular disease", *Canadian Cardiovascular Society position statement, Canadian Journal of Cardiology*, vol. 222, no 11, 2006, p. 913-927.

Alice H. LICHTENSTEIN, DSc. Chair FAHA, & al. "2006 Review of the recommendations for diet and health style living", *Scientific position of the Nutritional Comity of the American Heart Association, Circulation*, vol. 114, 2006, p. 82-96.

NATIONAL CHOLESTEROL EDUCATION PROGRAM EXPERT PANEL ON DETECTION, "Evaluation and treatment of high blood cholesterol in adults", *Adult Treatment Panel*, vol. 111, 2001.

HÔPITAL LAVAL, INSTITUT UNIVERSITAIRE DE CARDIOLOGIE ET DE PNEUMOLOGIE, Dietetic service, "Critères de Sélection pour le choix d'aliments Santé", "Comment déchiffrer les Étiquettes Nutritionnelles", "Les Fibres solubles, les Fibres insolubles", "Les Oméga-3", "Alimentation au restaurant", "Anticoagulothérapie", "Trucs de substitution pour améliorer vos recettes".

DIONNE, Johanne Dt.P., Mélissa LAGACÉ, Dt.P. "Anticoagulothérapie, uniformisons notre enseignement" in *La Nutrition, un élément essentiel en santé cardiovasculaire*, Institut Universitaire de Cardiologie et de Pneumologie, Hôpital Laval (May 2005).

CYR, Josianne Dt.P, "La vitamine K et les médicaments anticoagulants", dans *Nouveaux plaisirs de la cuisine santé*, Trécarré, 1997, p. xix-xx.

COLLECTIF, *Maigrir, la santé avant tout! Comment? Pourquoi? Pour qui?*, Les Éditions Protégez-vous in collaboration with L'Ordre Professionnel des Diététistes du Québec and "Équilibre", 2006.

DIABÈTE QUÉBEC, SANTÉ ET SERVICES SOCIAUX QUÉBEC, *Food Guide for the Diabetic person*, 2003.

BECEL, Becel Center for Heart Health: www.becel.ca.

BLAIS, Chantal Dt.P, Claude JOBIN, Dt.P, Émilie RAYMOND, Dt.P, Huguette-Andrée THÉRIAULT, Dt.P. *Mon guide nutritionnel pour prévenir et traiter l'hypertension artérielle*, Société québécoise d'hypertension artérielle, Montreal, 2005.

Bien acheter pour mieux manger, Les Éditions Protégez-vous, 2004.

HEALTH CANADA *Eating well with Canada's food guide*, 2007

Heart and stroke foundation of Québec: www.fmcoeur.ca

Centre de documentation sur la nutrition humaine: www.extenso.org.

American Heart Association: www.americanheart.org.

Acknowledgements

A project as ambitious as this one could not have been realized without the close collaboration of a number of people.

First, sincere thanks to Madame Margot Brun Cornellier and her family for having assisted our team, Louise Gagnon RD. M.Sc, Odette Navratil, RD M.Sc. and myself, in the creation of this valuable book.

Very special thanks to Madame Nicole Dubé at the Sandoz Canada Hospital Division, who supported me throughout the project with her wise advice, humanity and communication skills, and to Mesdames Louise Gagnon and Odette Navratil, my dietician/nutritionist collaborators, who shared their expertise and helped me revise the recipes and instructional document. Without the involvement of these three people, the project could never have come to fruition.

A document such as this one would not have been possible without financial assistance and a large-scale view of individual health; sincere thanks to Mr Gordon Meyer of the Sandoz Canada Hospital Division, a visionary who believed in the project. I cannot neglect to mention the Marketing team from Sandoz Canada, who gave me reinforcement at every step of the way, especially Mrs. Josée Lavoie, Product Manager, Marketing and Business Development.

My thanks also go out to Mr. Jean Francois Marsolais, dietician/nutritionist, for revising the recipes, calculating the nutritional values and diabetic exchanges, and to Madame Chantale Martineau, dietician/nutritionist, for revising the "Diabetes" section, and Madame Marie-Claude Vohl, PhD in Nutrition, for revising the item entitled "Nutrigenomics" in the "Cardiovascular nutrition – new developments" section.

Sincere thanks to Dr. Claude Gagné, former chief of Lipidology at the Centre hospitalier universitaire de Québec and Madame Roxanne Guindon, nutritionist and former team head for "Prevention and promotion" at the Heart and Stroke Foundation of Québec, for having agreed to revise the manuscript and for their invaluable advice.

All my gratitude goes to Doctor Paul J. Lupien, M.D., PhD., FRCP, FACB, FAHA, Founder and Director (1969-1995) of the Lipid Research Center, Laval University Hospital Center, for the revision of this English edition.

Last but not least, I wish to express my gratitude to those people who are dear to me and who accompanied me for the entire process: my friends, especially Thérèse Fournier and Thérèse Martel, my children and their partners: Anne-Marie, John, Yvan, Caroline, Richard, Isabelle «a culinary expert» and my grandchildren for their dynamism, which spurred me on, particularly my grandson Andrew for his unstinting encouragement.

THANK YOU!

Thérèse Laberge Samson, RD., nutritionist

Dear readers,

Since its creation, the mission of Sandoz Canada Inc. is to be a leader in health. As such, Sandoz preoccupies itself with the well-being of all Canadians and relentlessly contributes to it.

Sandoz currently commercializes over 85 molecules, many of which are used for treating cardiovascular diseases, hypercholesterolemia, hypertension and diabetes.

Marketing these medications is one of the ways in which Sandoz contributes to the well-being of Canadians. Financial participation in the publishing of "Your Health at Heart" is another way for Sandoz to encourage Canadians to take care of their health.

The constant increase in the use of non pharmacological methods in the treatment of such diseases shows that Canadians who are directly or indirectly affected by them are seeking complementary solutions to drug therapy. It is a privilege for Sandoz to provide its financial support to this project.

Bon appétit!

Pierre Fréchette
President & Chief Executive Officer
Sandoz Canada Inc.

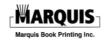

Marquis Book Printing Inc.

Québec, Canada
2009